FLOW

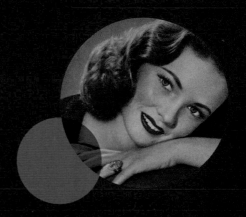

FLOW

THE CULTURAL STORY OF MENSTRUATION

Elissa Stein and Susan Kim

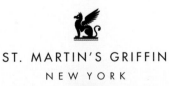

ST. MARTIN'S GRIFFIN
NEW YORK

FLOW. Copyright © 2009 by Elissa Stein and Susan Kim.
All rights reserved. Printed in China. For information,
address St. Martin's Press, 175 Fifth Avenue, New York, N.Y. 10010.

Production manager: Adriana Coada
Book design by Headcase Design

www.stmartins.com

Library of Congress Cataloging-in-Publication Data

Stein, Elissa.
Flow : the cultural story of menstruation / Elissa Stein and Susan Kim.—1st ed.
p. cm.
ISBN 978-0-312-37996-4
1. Menstruation—Social aspects. I. Title. II. Kim, Susan, 1958–.

QP263 .S73 2009
612.6'62—dc22

2009017046

First Edition: November 2009

10 9 8 7 6 5 4 3 2 1

To Jon and Heather, whose endless patience and support made all the difference.
And to Izzy and Jack, who challenge and inspire me every day.

—*Elissa Stein*

~~~~~~~~~~~~~~~~~~

To Lar, who always understands; to Ollie, who always listens; and to Evelyn, Melody, and Katie, who occasionally let me win.

—*Susan Kim*

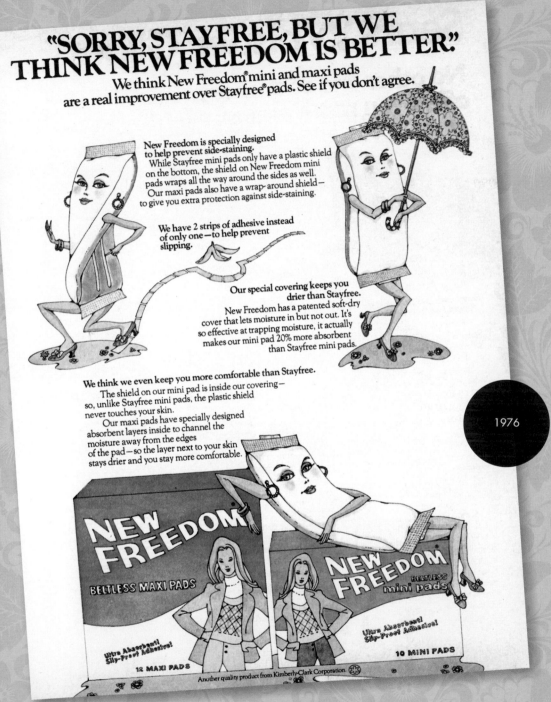

Contents

Introduction

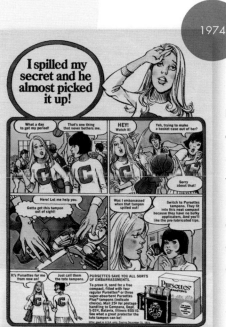

1974

FEMALES MAKE UP MORE THAN HALF of the world's population. And at some point, every single one of us, all 3.5 billion—pop stars, housewives, nuns, Masai tribeswomen, journalists, psycho killers, geisha girls, the queen of England, rocket scientists, cheerleaders, congresswomen, bag ladies— gets a regular period that lasts up to a week, about once a month, for forty years of our lives.

So why is menstruation still the ultimate taboo subject?

Swaddled with more superstitions and nontruths than Bigfoot, menstruation remains hidden in a figurative box (scented, of course), stuffed deep inside the great medicine cabinet of American culture: out of sight and unmentioned. Although this may explain why some of us still think it's dangerous to wash our hair during "that time of the month," there are spookier issues afoot. While we've been busy skirting the subject like the ladies we are, did you know that PMS—premenstrual syndrome—has been quietly labeled a mental disorder by the American Psychiatric Association? Or that there are still cases of Toxic Shock Syndrome every year? (Hey, didn't someone take care of that already?) Or that most tampons contain bleach and traces of dioxin? Or that there's a serious corporate campaign nationwide to abolish periods altogether?

Is any of this good? Is it bad? How can we figure out what to do when we can't even talk about bleeding in polite society?

Flow tells you where it's at when it comes to menstruation—what it is, what we've been told and how we've been sold, and what we should definitely know. It's the most natural of cycles with the most unnatural of histories. It's a funny, fascinating, and occasionally scary story of big business, advertising, feminism, gender roles, medicine, religion, world cultures, and, above all, *good manners* . . . in which every single female, young or old, will recognize her story.

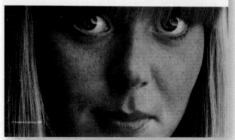

If you had an "accident" with your maxi pad last month, you're not alone...

Ever since I was a girl, it seems my period picked the wrong day to arrive.
Like the day I took my geometry final.
The night of my senior prom.
A job interview.
Not that I'm really complaining. But recently, on my way to my high school reunion, I could have done without my period.
The reunion was in Hadley. Quite a distance from the small New England town where I live. And wouldn't you know there was a traffic jam in Worcester. By the time I arrived, it had been a while since I left home. Then I remembered I had my period.
I raced upstairs to the powder room. I'd had an accident alright, but only my slip and I knew.
That's what made me try beltless Kotex maxi pads. Right on the back of the package how they have 13 absorbent layers. 13 absorbent layers sounds like a lot less chance of an accident. Especially when there are 3 adhesive strips to keep the pad in place.
If you had an accident last month, you owe it to yourself to try beltless Kotex maxi pads. Because accidents shouldn't happen. That's why I switched.

Kotex maxi and mini pads. Because "accidents" shouldn't happen.

Kimberly-Clark

It's all reinforced by menstruation's most devoted (you could say *only*) suitor, still faithful after all these years: the so-called feminine hygiene industry. Even though commercial menstrual products have been around for less than a century, they've meant big money from the word go. The industry's products, packages, messages, and advertising serve as a peculiar, frequently hilarious, and downright bizarre time line of all that's changed—and all that hasn't.

We're two women who, like all women, consider ourselves experts when it comes to our own periods . . . yet are paradoxically still full of uncertainties, questions, superstitions, and repressions. At the same time, we both pretty much take our periods for granted. For us, our periods are mildly inconvenient and reassuring at the same time: the uterus saying "all's well."

But is it really that simple?

The fact is, women in the twenty-first century menstruate a *whole* lot more in our lifetimes than we ever did before, since the beginning of recorded history. We eat better and weigh more, so we hit puberty younger. Our life expectancy has gone up, so we no longer routinely

no revealing outlines . . . but the same thickness, the same protective area

1933

Procter & Gamble Company

the new Phantom* Kotex

SANITARY NAPKIN
(U. S. Pat. No. 1,857,854)

...NT to eliminate those tell-
...es. Yet you must have safe,
...nitary protection. And that
... that . . . is what the new
...Kotex gives you.

...new design flattens and
...ends of your protection so
...without the tiniest reveal-
...e, yet the protective thick-
...*...tially* the same.

...ex features retained

...Phantom Kotex is in every
...ective as the Kotex you
...t, even after hours of use;
...y absorbent; disposable.
...itals alone more than 24
...tex pads were used last year.
...proved Kotex is brought
...ncrease in price. Never in
...has Kotex cost you so little!
...e confused. Other sanitary
...g themselves form-fitting
... sense the same as the
...tom Kotex, U. S. Pat. No.

...protection, each end of this
...om Kotex is now plainly
stamped "Kotex." It is on sale at all
drug, dry goods and department stores.
Also in vending cabinets through the
West Disinfecting Company.

HOW SHALL I TELL MY DAUGHTER?
Many a mother wonders. Now you simply
hand your daughter the story booklet entitled,
"Marjorie May's Twelfth Birthday." For free
copy, address Mary Pauline Callender, care of
Kotex Company, Room 2180A, 180 North
Michigan Avenue, Chicago.

Note! *Phantom Kotex has the same thick-
ness, the same protective area with the
added advantage of tapered ends.*

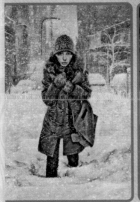
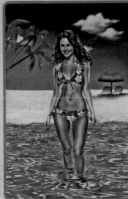

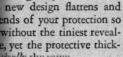
Upgrade!

Upgrade your life! Upgrade to Tampax Pearl!
With three fabulous details, it's our best protection ever!

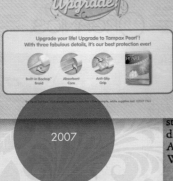

Built-in Backup™ Braid   Absorbent Core   Anti-Slip Grip

2007

Kimberly-Clark

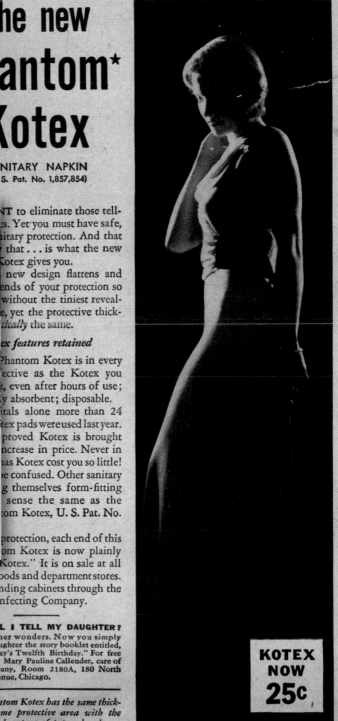

KOTEX NOW 25c

Copyright, 1933, Kotex Company

drop dead at forty. And unless you belong to some kind of cult, chances are you are not bearing and breast-feeding babies every second of your entire reproductive life, thus suppressing menstrual flow. If you add it all up, this means that you, Average American Female, will have something like five hundred periods in your long and lovely life. What does all this bleeding mean for us when it comes to our health? What does it mean about the products we buy to control the flow, and how does disposing of them affect the environment?

But what happens when your period doesn't play out like a tampon ad?

We know lots of women who, from their veiled hints and jokey complaints, appear to have a far more adversarial relationship with their periods than we do: irregular cycles, bad cramps, heavy flow, hellacious PMS, bloating. At the same time, no one we know actually discusses any of this openly, in any real detail. While it's apparently okay to share your political beliefs with a total stranger or post naked pictures of yourself on the Internet, divulging straight-faced details of your last period is still considered the ultimate faux pas.

But what happens when your period doesn't play out like a tampon ad? What if you secretly have real questions?

- What if you mysteriously stop menstruating even though you're young and definitely *not* pregnant?
- What if you're forty years old and find yourself beset by a monthly Red Tide lasting two weeks at a time?
- What if you start to bleed on a camping trip and are secretly convinced you're going to get eaten by a bear?
- If you're on the Pill, did you know that your monthly bleeding isn't even part of a real menstrual cycle at all? So what is it? Why is it even there?

- What *really* happens if you, heaven forbid, forget to remove a tampon at the end of your period?

- What about sex during your period? Is it gross? Dangerous?

- What did women use before tampons and pads were invented?

- What if you're approaching menopause and find you're deeply depressed? Or wildly exhilarated? Or spaced out like a zombie? Is something wrong with you?

- If it's true that a single disposable diaper takes approximately two million years to decompose, what's the story with all those used pads and tampons?

- Which is worse, when your boyfriend dismisses your occasional, plate-smashing fury as PMS or when he refuses to acknowledge there's actually something physiological going on?

- What if you're still not sure whether to use pads or tampons? Are there any other options out there? Are they safe? Are they sanitary?

- And what about period extraction? Is that a creepy 1970s thing or an actual option?

- What about chemically shortening periods with the Pill or stopping menstruation altogether? Is it safe? Is it a good idea? Would you miss it?

- Are there any women who still douche? Should you?

- What do other women do about all this? How do they feel?

- *What's normal, anyway?*

Over the years, we've both struggled with many such questions about our bodies and their cycles. As kids, we pored over the pamphlets that were covertly handed out in fifth grade or were stashed away inside the tampon boxes. As adults, we've talked to our gynecologists, we've read books and scoured the Internet, we've read political tracts about toxic shock and the Pill, we've browsed women's magazines and the alternative press about rumors and remedies, and we've traded anecdotes and complaints with our friends. But we couldn't find a single book that we as modern women could relate to: one that was supportive, informative, and honest. A book that we could share with the women and girls in our lives.

And that's why we wrote *Flow*.

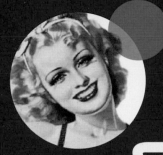

FLOW

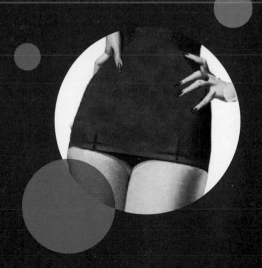

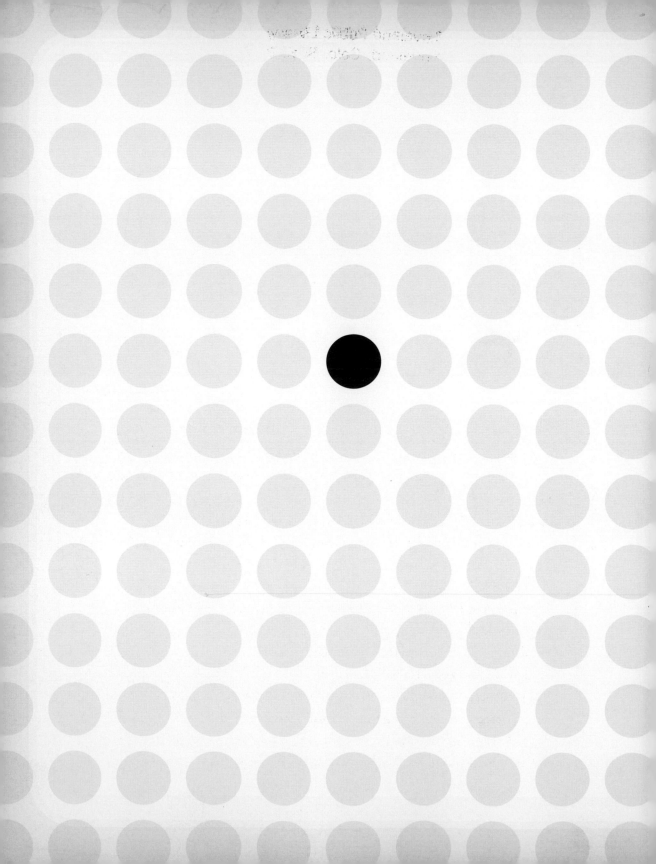

Chapter 1

LANGUAGE

FOR YEARS, FEMINIST SCHOLARS COMPLAINED BITTERLY that menstruation was a taboo subject in the United States. Back in the 1970s and early 1980s, you could hear the dark mutterings in women's health collectives and alternative bookstores across the country: Society kept any serious discussion of a woman's monthly cycle locked away in a figurative hut of superstition, sexism, and ignorance, far away from men, children, and the rest of polite society.

But of course, that was then, this is now. These days, what subject *isn't* talked about in broad daylight, right out loud—not only at home and at work, but on TV, in so-called family movies, on your very computer as you sit there innocently surfing the Web? It's quite possible, in one not very exciting day at home, to stumble upon detailed descriptions and actual videos that explicitly refer to not only menstruation but numerous other bodily parts and functions that would make even your hard-boiled, tough-talking Aunt Freida blush.

Menstruation is *everywhere!* Why, in 2007, they even ran a nationwide commercial promoting menstrual suppression right before the Oscars, for Pete's sake! Check out the commercials on daytime programming, pick up any magazine aimed at women or teenage girls. It's like the tampons and pads are practically leaping off the screen

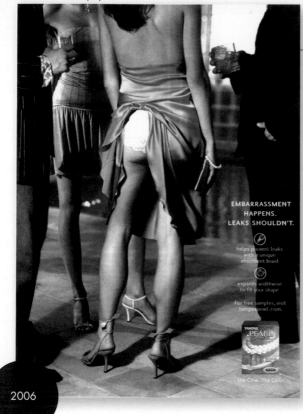

EMBARRASSMENT
HAPPENS.
LEAKS SHOULDN'T.

helps prevent leaks
with a unique
absorbent braid

expands widthwise
to fit your shape

For free samples, visit
tampaxpearl.com.

TAMPAX
PEARL

The One. The Only.

2006

and out of the pages to get at you! If there really was any kind of taboo against menstruation, it's a thing of the distant past, isn't it?

Well, yes . . . and no.

The catch—and it's a big one—is that whenever menstruation is mentioned these days, it's only because there's an underlying sales pitch. Either that, or it's the subject of a complaint or the punch line to a joke. Or all of the above. There's no real discussion of the actual event itself—not just the physiology and hormones of menstruation, but its complex history, its place in society, the inescapable role it plays in every woman's life, and its ramifications for our health, the environment, and our lives. (And we're sorry, no matter what any fifteen-year-old tells you, vulgarity alone does *not* count as honest discourse.)

The sad fact is that menstruation—the process, the images, the word itself—is as unspeakable and undercover as it ever was. Think about it—even in movies, TV shows, and commercials that actually mention menstruation by name, you never, ever see any sign of it. In fact, although you can watch buckets of fake blood merrily sploodging out of heads and torsos because of fists, bullets, knives, car accidents, grenades, bombs, breaking glass, garrotes, machetes, falling buildings, swords, laser beams, airline crashes, or hungry mutant zombies, rarely will you ever see a single drop as a result of menstruation. In 1995, a *Village Voice* cover featured a tasteful photo of a naked woman in profile, with a white string nonchalantly dangling between her thighs (the article was on Toxic Shock Syndrome), and from the subsequent outcry from readers, you would have thought the paper had endorsed Satan for president. (And this is the

Village Voice we're talking about, the paper that has routinely covered everything from genital piercing to golden showers.)

Even in the most up-to-date print ad or TV commercial, you will never once see a menstrual product being unwrapped, applied, inserted, tugged at, yanked out, pulled off, wadded up, wrapped in toilet paper, flushed, or thrown away—God forbid showing a before-and-after shot of a tampon (now that's a memorable visual!) or what it looks like when you accidentally spring a leak. The ads don't even show the inside of a bathroom, which is weird, considering that's where most tampons and pads are inserted or applied in the first place.

Whenever menstruation is mentioned these days, it's only because there's an underlying sales pitch.

The accompanying ad copy is invariably as bloodless as the images—neutral, soothing, and maddeningly vague. You can stare endlessly at a print ad featuring a beautiful woman walking across a field in a flowy gown, ponder the tagline "fresh, free, and natural" until your head feels like it's going to explode, and still come away not knowing what the hell they're selling: Is it air freshener? A new line of hemp clothing? A time-share in the Poconos?

The first time the word "period" was even mentioned in the entire history of TV advertising was in a Tampax commercial starring, funnily enough, Courteney Cox Arquette—and that

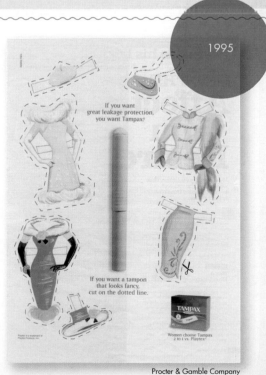

1995

If you want great leakage protection, you want Tampax.

If you want a tampon that looks fancy, cut on the dotted line.

TAMPAX

Women choose Tampax 2 to 1 vs. Playtex.

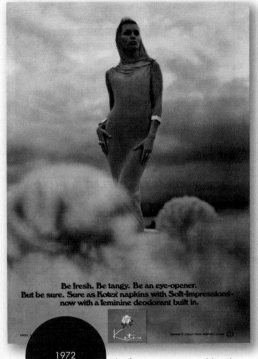

Be fresh. Be tangy. Be an eye-opener.
But be sure. Sure as Kotex napkins with Soft-Impressions—
now with a feminine deodorant built in.

Kotex

1972

wasn't until 1985! The Red Dot campaign by Kotex was the first to use the words "period" and "red," and that rabble-rousing piece of subversion didn't even occur until 2000.

Yet despite the ad world's contorted attempts not to show or say anything that could be seen as even remotely scandalous or off-putting, their efforts are apparently still not enough for most people. From what we can tell, public attitudes haven't changed much at all over the decades; as a result, menstrual ads have remained so incredibly sterilized and unspecific, you could look at them and honestly not even realize human blood was involved.

And it's not just a problem with advertising.

Our language itself has essentially been ...ed of menstruation, like there's been some kind of creepy propaganda campaign ...cing us to discuss it (if we do at all) in a mysterious code known only to CIA operatives. If you don't believe us, take a moment to consider the many, many ways we all refer to menstruation.

You're on the Rag. Your Friend's in Town, or maybe it's your Aunt Flo Who's Come to Visit, or your Aunt Ruby, or, for the sports-minded, the Red Sox Have a Home Game. Expressions for menstruation range from the jaunty (Saddling Up Old Rusty, the Tomato Boat Has Come In, a Visit from Cap'n Bloodsnatch) to the descriptive and occasionally gross (the Bleedies, the Dam Has Burst). There's also the essentially grim and resigned (the Curse, the Crud, the Misery, Monthly Trouble, the Nuisance, Being Unwell, Out of Commission).

Hey, it's always fun to complain, especially if it's about something inevitable (taxes, jury duty, that weird skin under your chin once you hit forty). Humor, after all, is the time-honored way we deal with discomfort, anxiety, and fear. What fits the bill

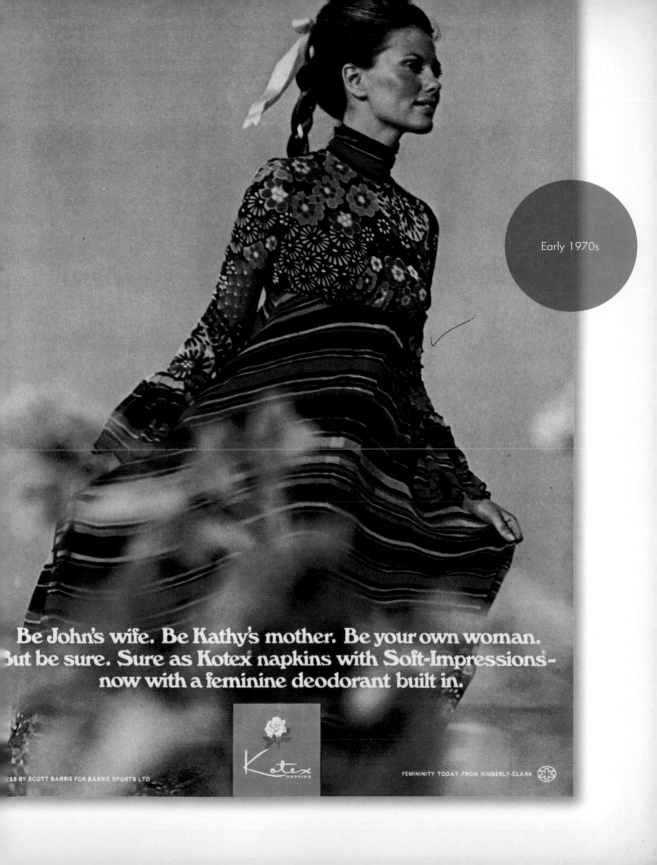

Early 1970s

Be John's wife. Be Kathy's mother. Be your own woman.
But be sure. Sure as Kotex napkins with Soft-Impressions—
now with a feminine deodorant built in.

Kotex
NAPKINS

255 BY SCOTT BARRIE FOR BARRIE SPORTS LTD

FEMININITY TODAY FROM KIMBERLY-CLARK

better than menstruation? Even if you're a perfectly well-adjusted, in-your-body kind of gal, who can resist telling her friends she's like Picasso in His Red Period or that she's Riding the Big Red Cadillac Down the Avenue of Womanhood?

There are creative film references for the pop culturists out there (Taking Carrie to the Prom, Miss Scarlett's Come Home to Tara), as well as endless uses of the word "red" (Code Red, Wearing the Red Badge of Courage, Off Visiting the Red Planet, Riding the Red Tide, Driving Through the Redwood Forest). If you're Having Ketchup with Your Steak, you might have to Walk Like an Egyptian or go Ram a Tam; if the Communists Have Invaded the Summer House, you probably need to go Change Your Cooter Plug or Straddle a Pad.

Look, we enjoy a good laugh as much as the next gal. Yet what freaks us out is that beneath all the bonhomie lurks the very real and unspoken message that as much as we're encouraged to make light about menstruation, we're somehow not supposed to be talking about it seriously. Is it just us, or don't you find it sinister when, say, a female lawyer in her thirties who can usually discuss anything from the G-8 summit to Etruscan pottery coyly lets slip that It's Arts and Crafts Week at Panty Camp?

And in case you were wondering, this isn't just the crazy, puritanical ol' US of A we're talking about here. Even those hip, sexy, sophisticated countries you think would be so *over* body shame have jokey expressions for the whole process. Worldwide, we've lost count, but we think there are currently about sixty trillion euphemisms for menstruation.

In the Netherlands, you might say *De Tomatensoep Is Overgekookt* (the Tomato Soup Is Overcooked); if you're Brazilian, it might be *Estou com Chico* (I'm with Chico); if you're Chinese, it's Little Sister Has Come; in Latin America, Jenny Has a Red Dress On; in Australia, I've Got the Flags Out; in Denmark, *Der Er Kommunister i Lysthuset* (There Are Communists in the Funhouse); in Ireland, I'm Wearing a Jam Rag.

People around the world have apparently taken to creative euphemizing with the zest of game show contestants. In England, there's I'm Flying the Japanese Flag (get out your Flags of the World placemat if this one eludes you); in Japan there's *Ichigo-chan* (Little Miss Strawberry); in France, *Les Anglais Sont Arrivés!* (The English Have Arrived, presumably in their traditional red coats). In Germany, it's *Die Waldbeerfrau Kommit* (the Cranberry Woman Is Coming) or *Ihren Kram Haben* (Have Your Trash); in Puerto Rico they ask, *¿Te Cantó el Gallo?* (Did the Rooster Already Sing?). In South Africa, Granny's

FIVE THINGS WE DIDN'T KNOW BEFORE WE WROTE THIS BOOK

1. **Your period on the Pill isn't really a period.**
2. **Doctors once stimulated patients to clitoral orgasms as treatment for hysteria.**
3. **Bloodletting came about to mimic menstruation, which was seen as a way to relieve bodies of noxious blood.**
4. **Hormone replacement drugs are made from the urine of pregnant mares.**
5. **There's a thriving menstrual porn industry.**

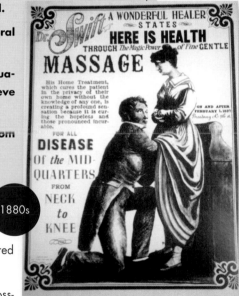

1880s

From a poster-size reproduction of an actual ad

Stuck in Traffic. And in Finland, PMS is charmingly referred to as *Hullun Lechman Tauti*, or mad cow disease.

Despite the humor and even the occasional grossness used to describe this most basic of female functions, what's actually taboo is any serious discussion of menstruation. If you don't believe us, just try this experiment: stroll into your next dinner party, family cookout, postwork happy hour—anywhere there's a reasonable mix of men and women, young and old—and try striking up a serious group conversation about, say, dioxin in tampons and its possible link to endometriosis. Watch as the faces around you swiftly turn to stone, as elderly relatives start to choke on the three-bean salad, as mothers whisk the kids away, as the menfolk get that strained look we know so well. Skirts will be drawn aside, and voilà! In a New York minute you will have become persona non grata.

Now, why is this?

We're not being annoyingly naïve here, so please bear with us. To you, this may seem like a weird question because the answer is so obvious. Nobody talks about menstruation because it's so, well, inherently distasteful. Plus, it's personal. Right? To many if not most women, a serious discussion about one's monthly flow in polite society is about as much of a conversational nonstarter as religion, how much money people make, and an in-depth analysis of one's genital warts.

Yet we have the sneaking suspicion that these seemingly unshakeable convictions of ours actually arise from centuries of calculated shame, moderated by money—with a dash of internalized objectification thrown in for good measure—as well as a genuine, centuries-old fear and suspicion of female body processes.

Paranoid? Who, us? Like flat-earthers laughing at crazy old Christopher Columbus who was so obviously about to go sailing off the edge of that ocean, many women may find it hard to believe that we all in fact have swallowed a line so completely that we can't even imagine life without it. And yet, bear with us a second as we mull this further.

In her book *The Curse: Confronting the Last Unmentionable Taboo: Menstruation,* Karen Houppert makes the point that even in these supposedly modern times, menstruation is always referred to with depressing, loser-ish verbs ("decay," "shred," "shrink," "slough," "disintegrate," "dribble," "discharge"), whereas ejaculation gets all the sexy, empowered, action-hero verbs (like "spurt," "spray," "pump," "shoot"). Be honest—with verbs like those, if you had to be a biological process, which would *you* rather choose? Even textbooks and gynecological literature make menstruation seem so, well, dweeby and passive: that what's *actually* going on, far from being the dynamic, incredibly complex process it is, is instead vaguely pathetic. We are left with the impression that the sad-sack uterus (pun intended) has once again not been asked to the pregnancy prom, so it just stays at home and lets it all go—that menstruation is, essentially, a lame combination of inertia and failure.

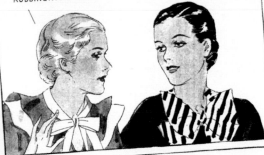

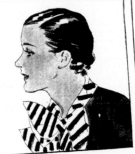

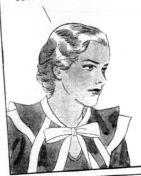

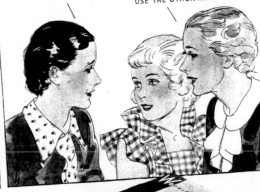

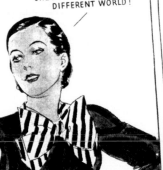

Here's new comfort...
NEW FREEDOM FROM EMBARRASSMENT FOR YOUR DAUGHTER

Most women think chafing is inescapable. But with this new Wondersoft Kotex you get about chafing entirely! Now sides are cushioned with fluffy cotton to keep them gentle, so downy-soft, that even young, vigorous of motion and tender of skin, find no fault. Sides remain dry and soft, top and bottom are free to absorb.

No twisting! No roping!

New Kotex constantly readjusts itself to conform to the body. Activities formerly impossible become pleasant. The special center gives even greater protection, offers safety against soiled lingerie.

Haven't you longed for just such a sanitary napkin as this? One that fits so snug that there are no telltale outlines under clinging gowns? Wondersoft Kotex is made for you women who want "forget-about-it" protection!...Buy Wondersoft Kotex at any store. Even the box doesn't look like an ordinary sanitary napkin package. And Super Kotex is now priced the same as regular size. In emergency, find Kotex in West cabinets in ladies' rest rooms.

Free Booklets!

Write for either or both of two authoritative booklets on Feminine Hygiene—"Health Facts on Menstruation"; and "Marjorie May's Twelfth Birthday", for a child. Address KOTEX COMPANY, Room 1430, 919 North Michigan Avenue, Chicago, Illinois.

ONE WOMAN TELLS ANOTHER ABOUT THIS NEW COMFORT

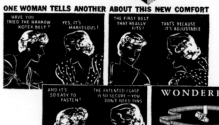

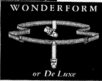

1930s

46
❧ *Refuse substitutes; buy the advertised brand every time!*

Language illustrates a basic tension: that people may talk about menstruation, but only when they reduce it somehow, dismissing it as the disgusting, eye-rolling nuisance everyone agrees it is. Periods are thus perceived as a dreary thing that happens to us—and not a complex and active process that is actually an integral part of our breathing, sweating, digesting, thinking bodies.

The underlying problem is something that the canny French philosopher Simone de Beauvoir put her nicotine-stained finger on in her groundbreaking 1949 book, *The Second Sex*: that in a world pretty much defined and dominated by men, women are seen as nothing more than the "other" sex, existing relative to the guys. Therefore, we stare with dismay at our own bodies, the way a landscaper might when faced with an especially unpromising patch of weedy, rocky, lumpy ground that must be ruthlessly weed-whacked into shape. Ever critical of the nagging unpredictabilities of our bodies, we're beset by anxiety, knowing we're supposed to be clean, dainty, and in control—and periods (All that blood and bloating! Those cramps! Such a temper!) are anything but.

So how does language fit into all of this?

In every conversation we have, the words we use to describe our bodies and their processes not only reflect but actually reinforce how we feel about them and how other people perceive them. This is why certain spokespeople get to go on the lecture circuit and make tons of dough talking about the power of positive talk . . . because it's actually *true*. The same is true for negative language. If, say, you decide to introduce a new proposal at the office with, "Here's another bad idea you're gonna think really sucks," chances are pretty good you've already shot yourself in the foot.

What makes all of this especially sinister is when we suddenly realize (like in our favorite scary story when the babysitter realizes *the killer is actually calling from upstairs!*) that the words we use, along with all their associations, have been already chosen for us years ago, in some cases even *centuries* ago. And by not questioning the words we've been programmed to use, we have indirectly absorbed their witchy power.

Consider the word "hysteria." A rampantly popular diagnosis for centuries, it comes from the Greek word *hystera*, or "uterus." The ancient Greek doctor Hippocrates (ca.

460 B.C. to 370 B.C.), normally such a swift guy that he was known as the father of medicine, seriously believed that the *hystera* was wont to wander around a woman's body. We're not kidding; he thought the uterus literally liked to mosey around a woman's torso, into her chest, and sometimes right up into her throat, in its never-ending search for children. Those ramblin' ways allegedly caused hysteria, a supposed illness that was still being diagnosed in women up until the early twentieth century.

In terms of language, there were no separate words for female genitalia for thousands of years. That was mostly because women were considered pretty much the same as men, only of course flimsier, more poorly designed, and incapable of writing in the snow. As a result, people used the same words to describe male and female organs: the ovaries were considered the female testicles, the vagina a penis, and so on. So how did anyone talk about menstruation, you might wonder? The answer: rarely, and in the vaguest possible terms.

Even today, advertisers and manufacturers tiptoe around the actual words, which are presumably too scary and horrible for our ladylike ears. Commercial menstrual products are commonly referred to as feminine "protection"; but this begs the question, protection against what? Against our big, mean uteruses and those psychokiller ovaries? Not to put too fine a point on it, but would you ever call a tissue "nose protection"?

Even the expression "feminine hygiene" implies that menstruation is fundamentally dirty, yecchy, bad, as does the expression "sanitary pad." Depending on your taste, menstrual flow may not be the most aesthetically bewitching substance you'll ever hold in your hand, but it's certainly not inherently unsanitary, either. Yet advertising, by continuing to refer to menstruation in such unrelentingly negative terms, reinforces the same message, over and over: that our monthly flow is a disgusting problem, a hygienic Three Mile Island, something so scary and awful that it *definitely* needs a solution. And don't worry, little lady: like a Fortune 500 knight in shining armor, guess who's volunteering to come rescue us from all that blood, that mess, our bodies?

In fact, menstruation isn't a Thing that just happens to poor, passive, slobby ol' us a few days every month for a few decades. It's actually a complex event, so much

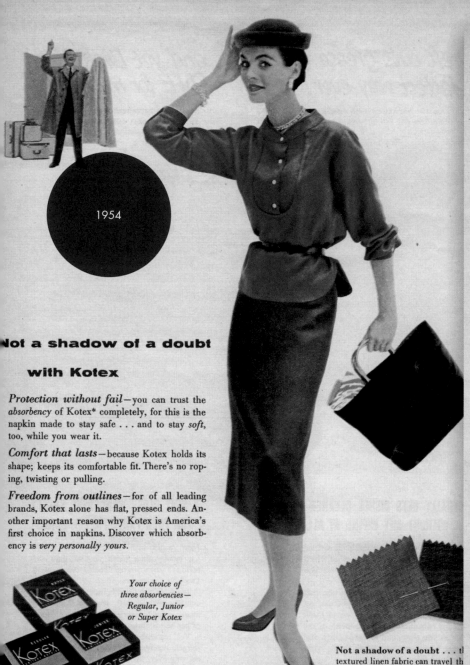

Not a shadow of a doubt

with Kotex

Protection without fail—you can trust the *absorbency* of Kotex* completely, for this is the napkin made to stay safe . . . and to stay *soft*, too, while you wear it.

Comfort that lasts—because Kotex holds its shape; keeps its comfortable fit. There's no roping, twisting or pulling.

Freedom from outlines—for of all leading brands, Kotex alone has flat, pressed ends. Another important reason why Kotex is America's first choice in napkins. Discover which absorbency is *very personally yours*.

Your choice of three absorbencies—Regular, Junior or Super Kotex

Not a shadow of a doubt . . . t... textured linen fabric can travel th... around. The separates, by Sportw... sun-warm colors: Capri blue an... green. Blouse about $10, skirt a... at leading stores.

More women choose Kotex than all other sanitary napkins

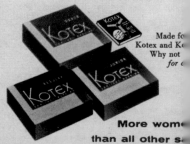

Not a shadow of a do...

with Kotex

Absorbency that doesn't fail—Kotex the trustworthy kind of protection you r... you get chafe-free *softness*, too, for Kotex to stay soft while you wear it.

Holds its shape—without twisting, ... pulling. That's why this napkin retains i... comfort for hours.

No revealing outlines—because only ... all leading brands has flat, pressed ends... important reason why Kotex is America's f... in napkins. Select the size best suited to... Regular, Junior or Super.

Made fo... Kotex and Ke... Why not ... for ...

More wome...
than all other s...

*T. M. REG. U...

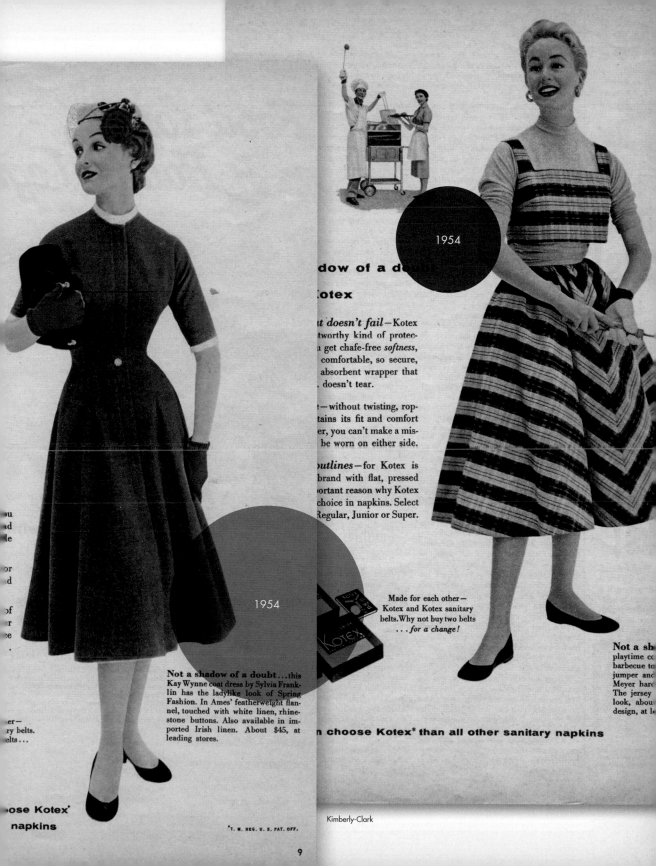

1954

Not a shadow of a doubt...this Kay Wynne coat dress by Sylvia Franklin has the ladylike look of Spring Fashion. In Ames' featherweight flannel, touched with white linen, rhinestone buttons. Also available in imported Irish linen. About $45, at leading stores.

...ose Kotex*
napkins

*T. M. REG. U. S. PAT. OFF.

...dow of a d...ubt

...Kotex

...t doesn't fail—Kotex
...tworthy kind of protec-
...a get chafe-free softness,
...comfortable, so secure,
...absorbent wrapper that
... doesn't tear.

...e—without twisting, rop-
...tains its fit and comfort
...er, you can't make a mis-
...be worn on either side.

...outlines—for Kotex is
...brand with flat, pressed
...portant reason why Kotex
...choice in napkins. Select
...Regular, Junior or Super.

Made for each other—
Kotex and Kotex sanitary
belts. Why not buy two belts
...for a change!

...n choose Kotex* than all other sanitary napkins

Not a sh...
playtime co...
barbecue to...
jumper and...
Meyer hard...
The jersey...
look, abou...
design, at l...

1954

Kimberly-Clark

so that doctors and scientists don't even fully understand it yet or what exactly it does. While it's true that most of us picked up the uterus-preparing-for-a-baby part by fifth grade, what we still don't know could fill a medical library. Only a few animal species on earth actually menstruate, humans among them. Why is that? How exactly is monthly bleeding tied to our health?

A big part of the problem is that, overwhelmingly, studies on menstruation tend to be funded by the "femcare" industry itself, and only, of course, to better develop and market their products. (As a rule of thumb, if you ever wonder about a particularly upbeat study plugging a product, just follow the money, honey! You'll find that, routinely, experts and pundits are quietly on the payroll of the companies whose products they're so enthusiastically endorsing.)

There have been more objective, scientific studies conducted over the years, but by and large, they tend to focus almost exclusively on the so-called pathological expressions of menstruation—not just the familiar downers like fibroids, endometriosis, and Lizzie Borden–esque PMS, but genuinely bizarro stuff (like the way women living together seem to bleed together, or when menstrual blood actually comes out of your nose).

Not to sound paranoid or anything, but we can't help but note that very few if any, science foundations, unive[rsities] and places of higher learning fran[kly give] a rat's ass about healthy menstr[uation.] The U.S. government itself created [the] National Institutes of Health's Office of

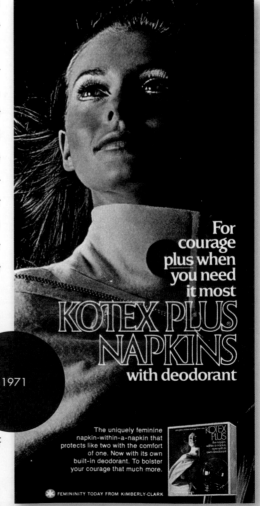

1971

For courage plus when you need it most
KOTEX PLUS NAPKINS
with deodorant

The uniquely feminine napkin-within-a-napkin that protects like two with the comfort of one. Now with its own built-in deodorant. To bolster your courage that much more.

FEMININITY TODAY FROM KIMBERLY-CLARK

Women's Health in 1990, and for a while, their single most burning question about menstruation was, "Does it make women unfit for combat?"

So where does that leave us? Totally in the dark? Screwed again?

Well, we do know some things, for certain. We know that for nearly all women, menstruation is a normal, if wildly variable and profoundly subjective, life experience. Another thing we know is that it seems to involve not just our uteruses, ovaries, and vaginas, but much of the rest of our bodies, as well: our brains, glands, hearts, and other organs. What's more, no matter how old we are, if we're female, we're actually menstrual our entire lives: either pre-, menstrual, peri-, menopausal, or post-. And the stages of our lives are in a sense defined by where we are on the menstrual time line.

Okay, we hear you demur. But why *talk* about it? We can envision certain relatives, friends, and colleagues pursing their lips en masse and rolling their eyes heavenward. "So this is what you want to talk about? With so much going on in the world, so many things to discuss, this is really so important?"

To which we reply: absolutely.

Recent studies show that up to 10 percent of girls still get their first period without any clue whatsoever as to what's going on (shower scene from *Carrie*, anyone?). What's more, college women consistently exhibit an amazing level of ignorance about the underlying biology of menstruation.

It's downright bizarre that what's called "discussion" about this most complex yet universal of processes has become one almost completely moderated by business and medicine. We've been taught our talking points by people who are frankly far more concerned with their bottom line than with any of those pesky questions we might have.

Hey, look—we're not saying that the pharmaceutical companies and femcare manufacturers are evil per se, or that their decisions are necessarily driven by some deep-seated misogyny or sexism. But business is business, and as of 2001, the so-called feminine hygiene business was a cool $2 billion industry—and that's just for the products themselves, not including related drugs or advertising.

Whether we're aware of it or not, our relationship to menstruation is one that has been brokered not in our own homes, but at the supermarket, the pharmacy, and the doctor's office. The conversation about menstruation (if you can call it that) is strictly one-sided and has been smoothly co-opted by big business, with a little help from religion, history, and society . . . and boy oh boy, do they have a lot to say.

So what can we do?

We can start by setting aside all the judgment and reexamining some of those crazy-making questions we've been ordered by society to be obsessed with since girlhood. (Do I smell? Does my pad show? Am I leaking? Did Harry from Accounting notice when the tampon fell out of my handbag?) How about we start asking other questions that are a lot more relevant to our lives today, like: Am I healthy? Is what I'm experiencing normal? Am I making the right choices for my body, my love life, my lifestyle, my planet? What's right for me? Am I teaching my daughters, my granddaughters, my kid sister good lessons about being a woman?

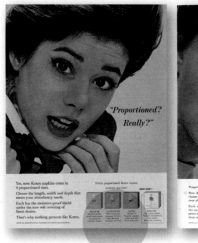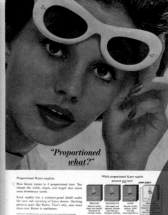

Enough with the ignorance and shame already! We say it's high time for a little more transparency. Let's perform a communal end run around the usual secrecy and embarrassment. Let's wrest control of this deeply personal topic away from the forces that have controlled it for so long. Armed with information and insight, maybe we can even figure out how to bring up the subject in polite company, without dying of mortification. Perhaps that way, we can spark a truly meaningful dialogue with ourselves, our friends, and our families about this most basic of functions . . . and how it affects us all.

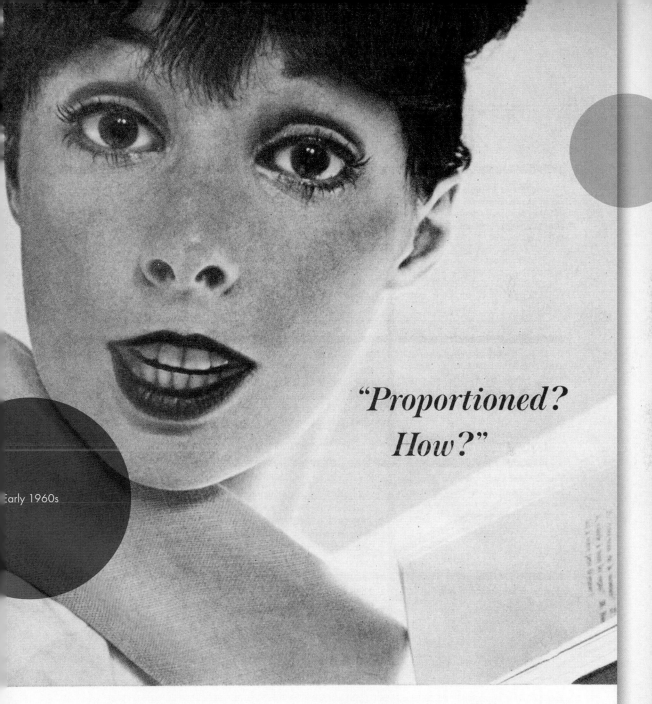

*"Proportioned?
How?"*

Early 1960s

Proportioned in width and depth as well as length.

Yes, now Kotex napkins come in 4 proportioned sizes so you can select the one that meets your special needs.

Each has the new moisture-proof shield.

That's why nothing protects quite like Kotex.

Which proportioned Kotex napkin protects y̲o̲u̲ best?

REGULAR	JUNIOR	SLENDERLINE	SUPER
Medium width, depth and length	Regular length and depth—less width	Narrowest, deepest, shorter than Regular	Regular length, deeper, wider

Now more than ever, Kotex is confidence.

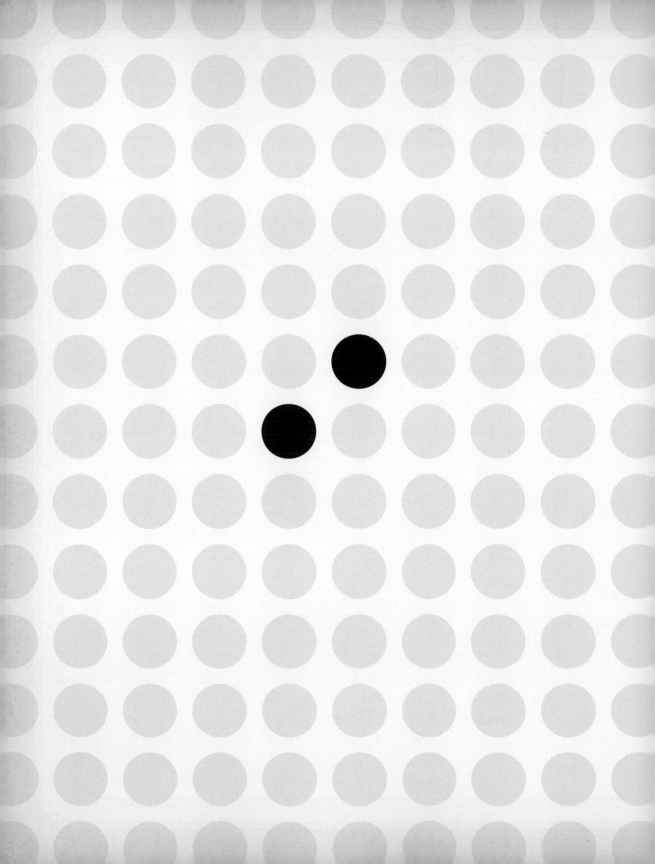

Chapter 2

WHERE WE ARE TODAY

SO HERE'S A PROPOSAL FOR YOU.
What if you could determine when, how much, and how often, if ever, you'd menstruate for the rest of your reproductive life? What if you could turn your flow off, not unlike a faucet, and then rev it back up again if, say, you ever wanted to get pregnant?

Sounds too good to be true? Well, pinch yourself, sister—your dream is now a reality, thanks to your pharmaceutical pals at Wyeth, Barr, Organon USA, Watson, Warner Chilcott, and Berlex Inc.!

"Menstrual suppression" is currently hovering like a multimillion-dollar question mark above our collective head, while countless scientists, advertisers, drug executives, gynecologists, femcare manufacturers, and shareholders wait breathlessly to hear how we're going to respond. It turns out that here in the twenty-first century, we seem to be poised on the threshold of a Brave New World when it comes to menstruation. The process itself is being chemically redefined in strange new ways, with all kinds of giddy promises being made and tantalizing possibilities dangled in front of our collective nose.

No more periods!

Who wouldn't be overjoyed, we're told by ads and articles that we're sure will only increase in number and shrillness as time goes by. What woman wouldn't love bidding adieu to all that mess, the cramps, the bloating? Who wouldn't want to get rid of the supplies, the black "just in case" pants with the stretchy waistband, the stained sheets and underwear, the painful breasts, the psychomeltdown PMS, the backaches? Why, no right-thinking woman alive, that's who! We're the lucky ones who get to live in an era when we can effortlessly pole-vault over our physical limitations to thrilling new heights of ease, comfort, and freedom. What kind of Neanderthal would knowingly choose to remain bound by her biology, imprisoned by the unthinking cycles of her animal self, stuck in an "imperfect" body?

Sounds like the answer is pretty obvious, right? And yet, we hesitate.

How many improvements can one make to a pad, anyway?

Don't get us wrong. We truly do appreciate that plenty of women flat-out hate their periods, and with ample reason. To them, menstruation is no friendly, gentle nuisance but a seriously painful, horribly messy, even health-threatening monthly event: a genuine curse. Even as women who don't have such negative feelings about our periods and are actually on pretty good terms with the whole process, we can certainly understand the appeal. If we can change the shape of our noses, vacuum fatty tissue from our buttocks, get a new kidney when one fails, correct blurry vision with lasers, fight killer infections with antibiotics, and have kids even if we're technically sterile . . . why shouldn't we be able to control our flow?

As far as we're concerned, part of our hearts leap at the glad thought of never again having to hand-scrub our underwear in cold water or beg another quarter off a stranger in a restroom just to buy an emergency tampon. And yet not to be wet blankets, when we consider the possibility of menstrual suppression, we are left more than a little confused, as well as downright concerned.

What disturbs us right off the bat is the one-size-fits-all assumption such a pitch is based on, since all of us have significantly different feelings about our periods. That which is unbearable to one woman is ho-hum and matter-of-fact to another; one woman's horrible monthly ordeal is another's womanly goddess ritual, and a vaguely irritating reassurance (I'm *not* pregnant!) to yet another.

Nevertheless, here we are, all being indoctrinated with the same line: that menstruation is so awful, of course we all want to get rid of it. What bothers us most is that the motives underlying this message are as suspect as they ever were, arising as they do not from hard science, long-term studies, or even from our actual needs or wants, but from the tender feelings of company shareholders.

So how did this all come about?

First, let's keep in mind that commercially produced femcare—pads, belts, tampons—has been around for only a hundred years or so. Since their launch, there have been noticeable improvements that we, for the most part, applaud madly. Who doesn't prefer that today's superabsorbent pads are wafer-thin, meaning that one no longer has to waddle around with the Manhattan Yellow Pages stuffed between her legs? Or that there's such a variety of tampon styles, sizes, and applicators, even a first-timer twelve-year-old can generally find something she can insert without the need for heavy sedatives?

And yet, even the most sanguine of businessmen realized long ago that there's ultimately a limit to what kinds of products can actually be made and sold to women when it comes to sopping up a few spoonfuls of blood every month. How many improvements can one make to a pad, anyway? If there's anything you *can* figure out about making a pad, say, even more absorbent, with even better wings, or perhaps an even prettier tampon with a glide-ier applicator, you can rest assured there are many teams of scientists feverishly working on it this very second. Yet dealing with the actual effluent of menstruation is just the tip of the revenue iceberg. Sure, there's money to be made from pads and tampons; but there's potentially huge money, *monster* dollars, to be harvested from tinkering with the actual process itself—something the medical community and pharmaceutical giants figured out years ago.

This all came about in large part due to one of the hottest trends that has sprung up over the past half century, one that sociologists in the 1970s dubbed "medicalization." Medicalization occurs when health or behavior conditions that have traditionally been thought of as being part of normal life are redefined by experts as actually being medical in nature—thus requiring medical solutions (e.g., drugs, surgery, hospitalization), as opposed to environmental, social, or even practical ones (e.g., a better diet, a raise in one's salary, more exercise, a full-time maid/cook/masseuse).

We're now experiencing a seismic marketing shift toward so-called preventive and quality-of-life drugs—medicines that treat an underlying condition. Invariably, the conditions are items on that vaguely dispiriting, seemingly endless list of what it means to be alive: sexual dysfunction, hay fever, obesity, bone thinning, restless leg syndrome, acid indigestion, even attention deficit disorder, depression, and anxiety. And yet all of these conditions have been systematically identified by the big pharmaceutical companies, who then developed the appropriate products, analyzed the proper markets, and pitched us, the lucky consumers. As a result, untold millions of dollars are now being made worldwide by treating conditions that weren't even identified as such for most of human history.

The catch is, medicalization is a complex subject that can't be solved by the simple equation "Drugs are bad, so just say no." We ourselves are not Luddites who are so antitechnology, we're still pushing mustard baths, mineral water purges, and homeopathic cures for serious underlying conditions. Nevertheless, what you don't know about the way pharmaceutical companies develop blockbuster drugs might give you serious pause.

If you were a giant company looking to make some major scratch by inventing a new drug, where would you start? First, you'd definitely steer clear of developing the cure to some weird disease (because not enough people contract it) or short-lived infections (because they don't last very long). No sir, in order for a drug to be insanely profitable, the potential market should be as big as possible . . . for example, "all women" is considered an excellent place to start. Furthermore, the ideal condition is something that, while annoying or even frightening, isn't going to progress so fast that it's going to kill anyone soon; it will hopefully linger on for years, ensuring a steady base of customers regularly holding aloft their prescription refills.

What fits the medicalization bill better than menstruation?

Patent and over-the-counter drugs to treat cramps and bloating have been around forever. Who doesn't remember covertly cadging a Midol off a girlfriend in junior high like it was contraband? Primarily made up of acetaminophen with a little caffeine and some antihistamines thrown in, Midol was heady stuff when we were teens. Today, of course, there are drugs out there that make Midol seem like a handful of jel-lybeans: Seasonale, Seasonique, Lybrel, Implanon, Yaz. Sounding like the lineup on some female sports team from outer space, these pills promise to reduce or even halt one's periods altogether for as long as one wants.

"But how can this be?" you may be exclaiming, falling to your knees from the sheer wonder of it all. "What sort of miraculous new drug are you talking about?" In fact, it's the same old wonder drug

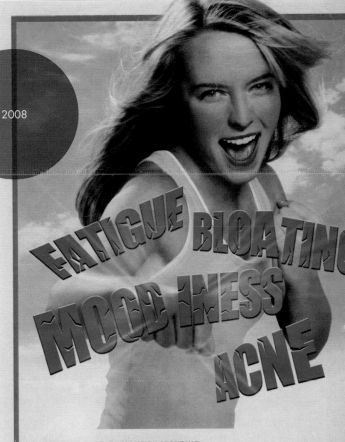

2008

IMPORTANT SAFETY INFORMATION ABOUT YAZ:
What are the risks involved with taking any oral contraceptive (OC)? OCs can be associated with increased risks of several serious side effects. OCs do not protect against HIV infection or other STDs. Women, especially those 35 and over, are strongly advised not to smoke because it increases the risk of serious cardiovascular side effects including blood clots, stroke, and heart attack.

Yaz, Bayer HealthCare Pharmaceuticals

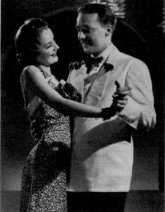
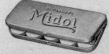
millions of us have already been taking for years and the single most common form of birth control here in the United States, constituting a $1.7 billion annual market. In short, menstruation suppressants are nothing more than birth control pills in a new package.

Regular birth control pills work in two ways: by thickening cervical mucus (which effectively prevents access to any eager-beaver sperm looking to hook up with an egg) and by flooding one's hapless body with synthetic hormones, effectively tricking it into thinking it's pregnant. As a result, ovulation ceases and the uterus stops building up its usual, heavy-duty layer of tissue, blood, and mucus.

"The Pill" actually consists of twenty-one active pills and a fourth week of placebos. When you take the placebos, the endometrium (which, due to the low-dose stream of synthetic hormones, has built itself up in a very half-assed way) breaks down and flows out. Once you start back up on the active pills, the uterus again builds up a fresh, skimpy lining. This explains why one's periods are not only light but incredibly regular when one is on the Pill. Everything is dictated by that precision flow of synthetic hormones.

One reason for building in this "pseudo-period" was that some pathologists were already worrying about the possible effects of a nonstop regimen of hormones. Another reason was that doctors felt that no period at all would be considered too freakish for most women to handle, and given what we know about 1960, the year the Pill came out, we think they were probably right. If you didn't perm your hair, wear a girdle, or go to bed with a fresh coat of lipstick, that practically made you a bongo-playing beatnik. What would anyone have made of menstrual suppression?

Sit down if this hasn't really sunk in yet, because this is the spooky part—*if you're currently on the Pill, that thing you've been calling your period all this time isn't one at all!* It's the Stepford wife of menstruation, in that it looks like a period and even kind of acts like one, but is ultimately not your period, plus is a lot better behaved and less argumentative. In other words, when you're on the Pill, your normal hormonal rhythms— that complex chemical symphony that controls ovulation, endometrial buildup, and flow—are essentially shut off. You're instead on an artificial merry-go-round of estrogen and synthetic progesterone, or progestin, which explains why there's less flow, no cramping, and virtually no PMS to speak of. It may look like a period, but technically speaking, it's not, at least not as any first-year medical student would define it.

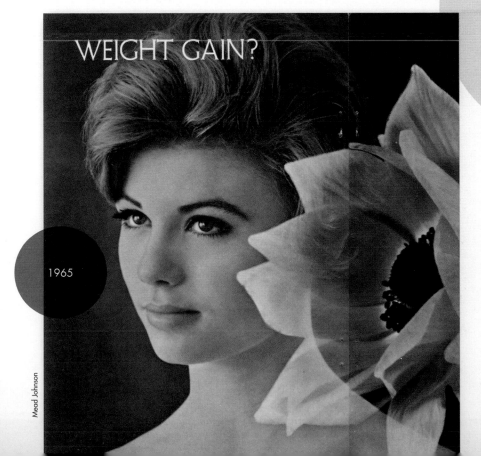

WEIGHT GAIN?

1965

Mead Johnson

ORACON®
16 White–Ethinyl Estradiol, 0.1 mg. Tablets; 5 Pink–Dimethi-sterone, 25 mg., and Ethinyl Estradiol, 0.1 mg. Tablets
THE FIRST SEQUENTIAL ORAL CONTRACEPTIVE

Offers your patients proven effectiveness plus these advantages:

1. Simulates the natural hormonal sequence
2. Simulates the natural endometrial response
3. Dramatically reduces breakthrough bleeding
4. Virtually eliminates amenorrhea
5. Lowest incidence of weight gain
6. Lowest incidence of first-cycle nausea

So why not take it a step further, wondered some shrewd scientist working late one night at some big drug company. What would happen if a woman just skipped that placebo week altogether?

According to the drug companies, this kind of menstrual management is the revolution American women have been waiting for all their lives. In a "clinical trial" paid for by the makers of Loestrin 24 Fe, 85 percent of the women polled said that "having their period" was one of their five greatest annoyances, along with "gaining weight" and "having a bad hair day."

Had we been polled, we perhaps would have written down "global warming," "unaffordable health insurance," and "the inexorable passage of time" as rating higher on the annoyance scale than our periods. We don't think we're alone on this one, either. Overwhelmingly, surveys not funded by drug companies have shown that most women simply don't consider getting their period that big a deal.

Of course, it's different for those who suffer from primary dysmenorrhea, endometriosis, fibroids, and the generic condition known as "bleeding like a stuck pig." Many have opted for the most radical way to ensure that they will never again menstruate: that is, they undergo a hysterectomy. Hysterectomy involves the surgical removal of one's uterus (with occasionally the cervix, ovaries, and fallopian tubes thrown in); and more than 600,000 are performed every year, making it currently the second most commonly performed surgical procedure in the United States. If you're currently considering a hysterectomy due to killer periods, the option of simply popping some pills instead may well seem like manna from heaven.

In May 2007, the FDA approved Lybrel, the first contraceptive formulated for the express purpose of eliminating menstruation altogether. True, up to 40 percent of the women in the test group were still experiencing breakthrough bleeding by the end of the one-year study, which we think kind of defeats the purpose. What's more, women found that not getting their period made it that much harder to realize they might in fact be pregnant, which can happen even if you're on the Pill. Yet this most likely didn't deter the champagne toasts and backslapping that went on the moment the FDA broke the happy news, and Lybrel landed on pharmacy shelves two months later.

Prior to their launch of Lybrel, Wyeth Pharmaceuticals commissioned a national study in which menstrual suppression (not surprisingly, considering that they paid for the study) got a thumbs-up from 97 percent of ob-gyns interviewed. Not only that, they reported other compelling statistics: women not only feel less effective during their periods, but take more sick days, avoid the gym, and wear dark clothes.

Overwhelmingly, surveys not funded by drug companies have shown that most women simply don't consider getting their period that big a deal.

Dark outfits and not working out? Well, why didn't you say so, man? This consti-tutes a national health emergency! Somebody, give those women a prescription for some expensive prescription drugs!

Come on, guys . . . can we have a reality check here? First of all, most women we know are already fond of dark clothing and don't work out, even when they're not menstruating. Furthermore, just because the drug companies appear to be stam-peding, lemming-like, over the cliff of menstrual hysteria doesn't mean that's a compel-ling argument for most women to follow.

What we'd really like to know is, how did this all come about? When did men-struation become such an outlaw, on the lam and apparently wanted by the FBI?

One of the most influential antimenstruation arguments made was in the 1999 book *Is Menstruation Obsolete?* Written by Elsimar M. Coutinho, the book was met with glowing reviews, as well as respectful, in-depth coverage by such tony publica-tions as *The New Yorker* and *The Guardian*. It claims that while many women insist on waxing sentimental about their periods, menstruation isn't the "natural state" it's cracked up to be. In fact, given the centuries-old tradition of women bearing and breast-feeding nonstop, Coutinho argues that regular periods are historically freakish, something that's only come about recently, as a result of less childbearing and nursing in developed countries, as well as improved overall health and nutrition. Far from being a healthy, even meaningful process, menstruation is a dangerous, biologically costly anachronism that places women at risk for serious medical and psychological problems, which the book then happily proceeds to recount in gory detail. In short, Coutinho makes the point that menstruation is pretty much an unnecessary evolutionary holdover, about as useful, meaningful, and natural as a vestigial flipper.

Coutinho is far from a crank; he's a respected professor of gynecology, obstetrics, and human reproduction. But he's also one of the pioneers of Depo-Provera, the injectable contraceptive that he endorses so strongly in his book. And while it can indeed relieve endometriosis, fibroids, anemia, and other problems, Depo-Provera is also linked to irreversible bone loss, as well as a delayed return to fertility afterward. For those unfortunate enough to accidentally become pregnant while using it, it's also linked to an 80 percent greater-than-usual chance of the child dying in his or her first year.

This, then, is yet another example of a widespread trend that can make a girl downright cynical: that far from being selfless and objective advocates of public health, doctors are more often paid spokespeople lurking in the pockets of the pharmaceutical companies . . . and take it from us, those are some *mighty* deep pockets. The pharmaceutical industry, after all, is routinely ranked as one of the top three most profitable businesses in the country.

As for their studies, we have good reason to question them. The big drug companies love nothing more than distinguished experts and academics writing them and their products up flatteringly in articles, speeches, and yes, books aimed at general readers like you and me. Talk about getting a Good Housekeeping Seal of Approval! The companies therefore woo such potential opinion makers madly with expensive gifts, hefty speaking fees, and exotic trips to faraway conferences. A 2003 editorial in *The Washington Post* summed up the conflict: "Anyone arguing the drug companies' case, no matter how neutral his or her academic or think-tank position may seem, should be questioned carefully with regard to sources of income."

The big pharmaceutical companies have thus spent huge amounts to make some pretty crafty arguments about why we should seriously considering shortening, reducing, or even ending our periods outright. When they're not creeping us out with medical horror stories, they pathologize the symptoms, demonize the event, and, ultimately, convince us to feel lousy about something that honestly shouldn't be that big a deal to most women. The National Women's Health Network recently reported on the increasingly negative way menstruation was being talked about in the world of health care and how it was subsequently spun by doctors to their female patients. By their reckoning, the propaganda is working all too well: there seems to be a spike in negative attitudes about menstruation, especially among younger women.

But what are the facts?

Is there in fact any truth to the many claims of those who endorse menstrual suppression? A woman will shed up to forty quarts of blood, mucus, and tissue in a healthy lifetime of menstruation, but to what end? What's the *point* of monthly blood, anyway?

Funnily enough, virtually no medical school, scientific think tank, or research lab had ever seriously studied this question until 1993. As of the twenty-first century, no one has yet been able to prove exactly why we menstruate and how it affects our health. One theory is that the shedding of blood every month acts as a built-in cleaning system that regularly tidies away any contaminating microorganisms, especially those brought in by sperm. Critics of that theory retort that microorganisms love nothing better than growing in blood. Still others chime in that the whole point of menstruation isn't about blood loss; the ongoing regrowth of the endometrium is just more cost-efficient than keeping it in constant running order.

Other theories abound. In her 1999 book, *Woman: An Intimate Geography*, Natalie Angier suggests that the human brain is so advanced, a developing fetus needs vast amounts of blood to feed it; therefore, the constant regeneration of the endometrium is actually a sound investment. Others argue that a fresh uterine lining every month, one that won't respond to an invading foreign body with an inflammatory response, is essential to prevent rejection of a fertilized egg.

Since various organs perform numerous chores (the humble liver is responsible for more than five hundred), some believe that the uterus, via menstruation, helps reduce our blood pressure and iron levels, thereby trimming our overall risk of heart attacks and stroke. Furthermore, it can be argued that our heart health is helped by the presence of estrogen, which lowers the "bad" kind of cholesterol while increasing the "good." Still others theorize that the hormonal shifts of menstruation are mysteriously linked to what we like to smell and how we ultimately choose our mates.

So little is actually known about menstruation that it's hard to predict what the unintended effects of widespread suppression might be.

So little is actually known about menstruation that it's hard to predict what the unintended effects of widespread suppression might be. And what of the drugs themselves and their long-term effect on our bodies? What exactly happens to us if and when we use hormones to stop our periods?

What freaks us out not a little is the extraordinarily skimpy testing that's been done on menstrual suppression to date. Barr Laboratories, for instance, claims that Seasonale is safe enough to take from one's teens all the way through menopause. But before you go rushing out to fill that prescription for your fifteen-year-old, do you want to know what this claim is based on? On a study of three hundred women who were tested for one year . . . total. To us, this is exactly not what we'd call reassuring.

Scientists from the Yerkes National Primate Research Center of Emory University and the Center for Behavioral Neuroscience in Atlanta conducted a study in 2007 on the synthetic progesterone used widely in contraceptives. They discovered that it made female monkeys more aggressive and anxious, while dampening their sex drives—not really an appealing combination for anybody. Obviously, this was only one study, but it might help explain reports of mood changes, heightened anxiety, depression, and loss of libido in women who use synthetic hormones for contraception . . . and conceivably for menstrual suppression, as well.

Another weird and disturbing long-term effect of menstrual suppression is actually environmental, and we're not even talking about the typical pollution you'd expect from industrial manufacturing. In recent years, there have been Stephen King–esque reports from the United States and England about animals that live in or near the water: male alligators with undersize penises, male fish that produce eggs as well as sperm, male sea birds with distinct hermaphroditic changes.

Sounding like the setup for a not-very-funny episode of *Futurama*, this state of affairs is most likely caused by synthetic estrogen from birth control pills. More than 100 million women worldwide are currently on the Pill; every day, they excrete vast amounts of leftover synthetic estrogen (which is more potent than the natural kind), which eventually makes its way to the nation's rivers and streams.

So what might this kind of unintended estrogen exposure do to humans, particularly the ones who eat fish? No one really knows yet, although there's already speculation that it might be linked to early puberty in girls, breast cancer in women, and decreased sperm count.

Could it be we simply don't have enough evidence to prove that menstrual suppression is reversible or even safe in the long run? While originally recommended only for women with physical problems such as painful endometriosis, suppression is now being hawked to everyone. The problem is that most of the women signing up are not the ones with actual medical conditions, but those who have negative attitudes about their periods, attitudes encouraged by the drug makers themselves. When it comes right down to it, is that really how we want to make decisions about our bodies?

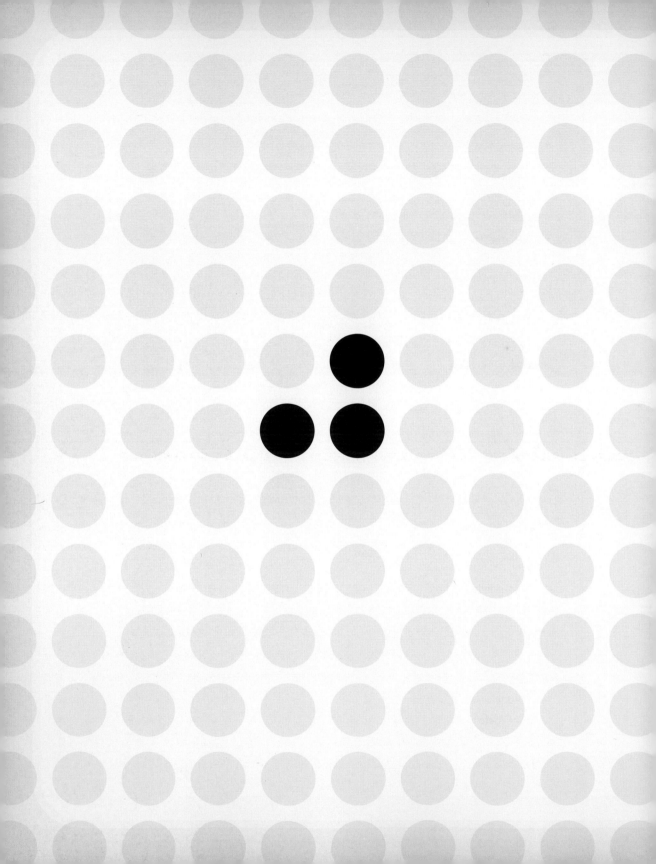

Chapter 3

SO HOW DID WE GET HERE?

SO HOW ON GOD'S SWEET EARTH DID WE GET here, anyway?

In a world beset by genuine problems, how did menstruation become the ultimate taboo? When did a woman's monthly flow become so unacceptable that vast amounts of time, money, and effort are now spent annually trying to thwart it? In short, how has the civilized world managed to get its collective panties into such a bunch about menstruation?

The answer isn't simply corporate greed, or scientific hubris run amok, or even that good old standby, American prudishness. In fact, to truly understand how and why menstruation became such anathema, one is compelled to look back—way, *way* back, thousands of years back, before the Discovery Channel, Charles Darwin, and Bill Nye the Science Guy.

Back before the concept of science was even articulated as such, people were compelled to come up with their own answers for all those pesky, niggly little questions that haunted their days. Why did the bright yellow ball appear in the sky every morning and disappear at night? Why did big, black woolly things fill the sky, let loose gouts of water, and occasionally go *boom*? Why did some green things taste good while others made you feel funny, lie down, and eventually stop breathing? And why did bright red stuff, the kind that came out of you when you were gored by a mastodon, ooze out of women every moon cycle, with no apparent harm done?

The way we see it, if you belonged to a people for whom the trickling of a river probably led to a great fear and lasting awe of the Water God, the ability to give birth to a living child must have seemed the most amazing, wondrous thing imaginable. And yet why did such a vast majority of ancient societies clearly look down on women, treating them as inferior beings? Why have the females, throughout history, consistently ended up with the hairy end of the lollypop?

Why have the females, throughout history, consistently ended up with the hairy end of the lollypop?

Was it because the women were usually hunkered down by the campfire, tending to the food and taking care of the offspring? Was it because the men were bigger, stronger, loaded with testosterone, and carrying the spears? Or was it all somehow triggered by that weird female bleeding? Was menstruation seen as some kind of imperfection? Some divine warning? A literal curse?

Whatever the reason, societies and religions sprang up worldwide that were overwhelmingly patriarchal, the hierarchy being invariably one that, surprise surprise, favored the guys. Being atop the social ladder not only allowed men all the advantages you'd expect, such as better access to goods and services, and greater freedom, it also put them in the position to create and reinforce myth. This, as you will quickly gather, was no shabby perk and may in fact explain why so many early religions and mythologies degraded, demonized, or simply ignored women—as if to pooh-pooh what must have seemed her eerily mystical power to create life. Just sling open your Old Testament, that bedrock of Judeo/Christian/Islamic faith. Right there in chapter 1, Genesis, God is most unmistakably male, a "he" with a capital *H*, and take it from us if you haven't read it recently, there's nothing even remotely feminine about that first week of creation. Yet long before the Bible was being laboriously etched on papyrus or carved on tablets, men had already set down complex stories about superbeings, gods and goddesses who were responsible for everything we pathetic mortals couldn't begin to fathom.

The good news is that the female goddess character was often described as possessing great power. The bad news is that it was invariably portrayed as a negative, destructive force, one that more than outweighed her ability to create, effectively turning her into a sort of cosmic Joan Crawford in *Mommie Dearest.* Such a storyline reinforced the notion that while women may be able to bring forth life, they're also responsible for everything awful that goes down afterward, as well.

Take the story of the goddess Tiamat, mother of ancient Mesopotamia, from Babylonian mythology. Tiamat is no mere goddess with a halo and a toga, but a horrifying, roiling ocean, a nightmarish embodiment of pure chaos. Flattering enough for you? She does manage to give birth to the first generation of gods, but must then be killed after she attempts a hostile takeover of the entire universe. Following this dubious model was Gaia, the incestuous Mother Earth from ancient Greece, who egged on her children to castrate their father/brother, Uranus. Then there's the Aztec goddess Coatlicue ("the one with the skirt of serpents"), who to this day is still portrayed sporting not only her distinctive outfit, but also a festive necklace made of human hearts, skulls, and hands. She embodied both birth and death, and her own children ended up having to kill her.

So how did menstruation figure into any of this?

Back before anyone understood the finer points of reproduction, people were nevertheless on to the idea that women occasionally stopped menstruating, their bellies grew bigger, and they'd give birth, after which the bleeding would eventually start up again. It didn't seem unreasonable to assume that the blood a woman retained during the swollen-belly stage was somehow transforming itself into a baby and that monthly blood was the residue of an unborn child. No wonder menstrual blood was both feared and considered sacred. Ancient peoples believed it was the very stuff that life came from.

This may explain why menstrual blood made its way into early mythology and became such an integral part of the story of creation. According to Hindu legend, when the Great Mother made the universe, her "substances clotted," thereby birthing the cosmos. And in biblical lore, the name of the first man in Genesis, Adam, comes from the Hebrew word *adamah*, meaning "bloody clay." Not surprisingly, the notion that the first man was somehow jury-rigged out of clay and menstrual blood didn't end up making it into the King James Version. Today, most biblical scholars cite instead a vaguer reference to "red earth."

Leaping sideways from early religion and mythology, we land squarely in the world of science and medicine and discover, unsurprisingly, that perceptions of menstruation weren't so enlightened there, either. Back in the 300s B.C., the great scientific philosopher Aristotle also concluded that menstrual flow was excess blood that hadn't yet been made into a fetus. Not that a woman actually created life; apparently, menstrual blood was inert and useless until it encountered semen, which added form and triggered fetal growth. To him, woman was basically just a passive receptacle, a container of gooey, formless matter that needed a man to bring order (namely life) to the chaos. What's more, Aristotle believed that while a woman contributed to the physical aspect of a baby, it was the man who gave it its soul.

To be fair to Aristotle and the ancient Greeks, their scientific and medical conclusions were seriously hampered not only by laws and religious strictures against dissecting human cadavers, but by prevailing sexism and unchallenged assumptions, as well. Male and female reproductive systems were considered mirror images of each other, with the female ranking a distinct second to the male. Monthly bleeding, after all, seemed to indicate the perpetual breaking down of tissue and was considered all but proof of a woman's inherent inferiority.

The poor old uterus itself was considered the underlying problem: the source of all that gooey blood, the root of woman's inferiority, and the cause of many, if not most, of her problems. In fact, the uterus was such a vivid presence to the ancient Greeks, it was literally assigned a character. Aristotle's teacher, the philosopher Plato, wrote, "The animal within them (the so-called womb or matrix) is desirous of procreating children, and when remaining unfruitful long beyond its proper time, gets discontented and angry, and wandering in every direction through the body, closes up the passages of the breath, and, by obstructing respiration, drives them to extremity, causing all varieties of disease."

Did you follow that? Plato wasn't being all figurative and poetic when he wrote that the uterus "wandered in every direction"; he, and countless others, believed that the womb was literally autonomous, a strange little critter that freely roamed around the female body, in search of children. It had feelings. And it could get lonely.

In a moment of perverse inspiration, Hippocrates, the so-called father of medicine, theorized that the uterus was in fact the source of female emotions. If one were unfortunate enough to possess a temperamental uterus that decided to go rampaging through one's body willy-nilly, this manifested itself as a condition called hysteria. This one notion turned out to be perhaps the ultimate gold star of misguided medical theories, a genuine keeper that lasted, horrifyingly enough, for centuries. But more on that later.

From the very beginning, ignorance about female anatomy and anxieties about sex built to a perfect storm of bizarre menstrual speculation. In A.D. 77, writer and philosopher Pliny the Elder wrote a thirty-seven-volume encyclopedia called *Natural History*, which included numerous hair-raising theories on menstruation. According to Pliny, menstrual blood could make seeds infertile, kill insects, kill flowers, kill grass, cause fruit to fall off trees, dull razors, and drive dogs mad. The glance of a menstruating woman could kill bees, her touch could make a horse miscarry, and contact with her blood would cause another woman to lose her child, as well. A menstruating woman could cloud a mirror, but, fortunately, fix it again if she stared really hard at the back of it. Pliny also advised men that sex with a menstruating woman during a full lunar eclipse was not only a bad idea, but a potentially fatal one.

Oh, those funny ancient Romans with their wacky, outdated ideas! The laughter, however, quickly dies on our lips when we take note that Pliny's theories didn't go officially unchallenged until 1492, more than a thousand years later. Many truly believed—still do, in fact—that menstrual blood was a poisonous, noxious substance that could wreak havoc on animals, plants, food, mirrors, and hapless men. As recently as the 1920s, menstruating women were barred from certain churches (since their very presence would defile the sacred place), from Mexican silver mines (since they'd cause all the precious metal to magically disappear), and Vietnamese opium labs (since they'd turn the drug bitter).

Funnily enough, even the word "taboo" relates to menstruation.

Similar prohibitions kept menstruating women far from food production, as well. In many countries, it was believed to be dangerous to eat anything prepared by a menstruating woman because her condition would poison the food. French sugar refineries felt she'd make the sugar blacken; German wine makers were convinced she'd make the wine turn sour; and in parts of England, it was believed a menstruating woman would spoil meat just by hanging around, innocently minding her own business. It was a given that the very presence of a menstruating woman would ruin a hunt. What's more, if a hunter were dumb enough to actually have sex with a menstruating women beforehand, the prey would somehow *sense* this and stay far away.

Funnily enough, even the word "taboo" relates to menstruation. It comes from the Polynesian word *tupua*, which means "sacred" and is also used when referring to menstruation. In fact, menstrual blood has historically been reviled as the most evil and poisonous of substances, while being strangely revered as sacred and powerful.

Counterintuitive, no? And yet in her 1996 *Encyclopedia of Myths and Secrets*, Barbara Walker writes that menstrual blood was often a valuable, integral ingredient in ancient rituals and ceremonies—both in mythology and in the real world—used for everything from an ingredient in wine given to Greek gods, to both a beverage and bath for fellow deities of the Hindu Great Mother. Imbibing menstrual blood, whether literally or symbolically, was clearly powerful stuff, and not just in the stomach-churning sense. It could confer immortality to Egyptian pharaohs, Celtic kings, and even early followers of the Tao.

And yet anything considered that powerful—plutonium, nuclear waste, menstrual blood—inherently carries at least the threat of danger, as well, and from it must invariably arise rules about its strict containment. For centuries and in numerous countries, this often meant being shut away in a "menstrual hut" during one's period, far from food, sex, and, presumably, pregnant horses, sugar and opium factories, mirrors, and wine makers.

So what do we make of this? Certainly, it can seem by today's standards like the ultimate gender diss, being forced into a dark hut and treated like some kind of leper for four days each month, in some cases being forced to use special utensils so no one could catch your cooties. But who knows? Even though your typical menstrual hut was apparently a far cry from a day spa, perhaps women actually appreciated the time off, a time when they could routinely escape the rigors of daily life.

Historically, menarche, aka the onset of menstruation, has had rituals of its own. In *The Curse: Confronting the Last Unmentionable Taboo: Menstruation*, Karen Houppert listed various charming menarche rites from the distant past. If one were a British Columbian Indian, one would have been secluded, in the wilderness, for three or four years running. The more civilized natives of New Ireland kept their girls at home for the same amount of time, but in cages, where they could be easily fattened up to better display the family's prosperity. The *really* rich families could afford to lock their girls up for years while they happily plumped them up, not unlike geese for foie gras. In other cultures, girls were variously kept under mosquito netting, buried in sand, or locked by themselves in tiny, dark huts. And even in supposedly civilized Western culture, upper-class adolescent girls were introduced to the painful rigors of corsetry, competitive coming-out seasons, and the unyielding societal rules that made all of Edith Wharton's heroines so damn miserable.

And yet, believe it or not, not all menstrual superstitions were unremittingly hor-rific. In many cultures, a young girl entering puberty was seen as cause for celebra-tion. Pliny the Elder reported that Greeks and Romans believed a menstruating woman could calm a tempest and rescue ships foundering in severe storms. That, friends, ain't hay. And remember how Pliny thought that a bleeding woman could kill insects? Well, in his words, "If a woman strips herself while she is menstruating and walks round a field of wheat, the caterpillars, worms, beetles, and other vermin will fall from the ears of corn." Talk about a green alternative to pesticides . . . or should we say red?

Hippocrates himself believed menstruation would "purge women of bad humors," bringing relief from headaches, nervous tension, and what sounds suspiciously to us like PMS. He also believed menstruation was the body's way of getting rid of excess blood that was responsible for imbalance and disease. As a result, he concluded that men would benefit if they were purged of diseased blood, too. The Greek physician Galen took Hippocrates' theory one step further and introduced regular bloodletting as both medical treatment and a way of balancing the blood, one of the four humors (along with yellow bile, black bile, and phlegm). He came up with an elaborate system of how much blood should be drawn based on an analysis of not only the patient's age, health, and symptoms, but also the season, weather, and location.

As lame as it sounds, "humorism" was actually the medical rage in Western culture until the 1600s; and even after it fell by the wayside, bloodletting remained popular for both sexes throughout much of the nineteenth century, including women who were menstruating or pregnant. After the medical community rallied to denounce the practice, Edward Tilt, a renowned London physician, defiantly published a book in 1857 in which he defended the use of bloodletting to treat menopause. He argued that since it mimicked menstruation (well, kind of), it would obviously cure hot flashes, headaches, and dizziness.

And do you know who the primary bloodletters were? Not physicians . . . but barbers. That iconic red-and-white striped barber pole symbolized both red blood and a white tourniquet; the pole itself called to mind the stick patients were asked to squeeze in order to dilate their veins. And did you know Mr. I-Cannot-Tell-a-Lie, George Washington, first American president and father of our country, most likely died due to some overzealous bloodletting? After falling ill, he was bled repeatedly the following day for a total of eighty-two ounces, the amount in almost seven cans of Coke. Not surprisingly, he died that night.

We can all breathe a collective sigh of relief that the more drastic theories and treatments of the ancient world disappeared like the morning dew in the past century as scientific discovery rendered them obsolete. And yet many superstitions about menstruation stubbornly lingered on. In a 1943 booklet put out by Kotex, "That Day Is Here Again," common superstitions of the day were listed in a section called "When Grandma Was a Girl":

> If she drank milk, the cows were doomed.
> If she entered a wine cellar, wine went sour.
> Flowers would wither away at her touch. . . .
> Meat would spoil if she dared to salt it.
> A look from her eyes would kill a swarm of bees.
> Clocks stopped during her period.

Did Grandma realize that many of her cherished superstitions dated back to Pliny the Elder, circa A.D. 77? The booklet quickly went on to debunk these myths, along with others involving bathing, shampooing, and exercising . . . but the fact that there were so many myths that actually needed debunking in the first place gives one serious pause. And despite their seeming step forward toward enlightenment, Kotex was quick to point out other limitations. They sternly warned menstruating women against imbibing cocktails—too much stimulation was bad for the system! They put a similar kibosh on swimming: sudden immersion in cold water could shock your system and stop your flow! In fact, any sort of physical overexertion was best avoided. And wet feet spelled potential disaster.

In his 1866 book, *Women and Her Diseases*, Dr. Edward Dixon also zeroed in on the wet foot problem. As he saw it, cold congested the uterus; sporting flimsy calfskin slippers on a chilly day would certainly be enough to stop menstrual flow. He disapprovingly mentioned patients of his, madcap girls who routinely soaked their

Thumbs Down —

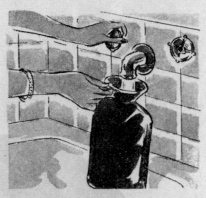

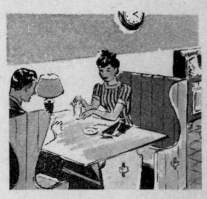

To douche, or not to douche? Certainly not on "those" days! Matter of fact, some doctors frown on any douching at all—*except* when prescribed for some special ailment. Trust your daily bath and deodorant to keep you dainty.

Cocktail-crazy? Tut, tut! Too much stimulation's bad at *any* time. "High" tonight—low tomorrow. (Nature drives a hard bargain!) And during menstruation, more than ever—that logy, let-down feeling's just what a woman needs everything else *but!*

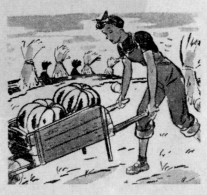

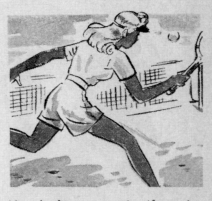

Carry on—but carry *lightly*. Don't tote more than you can manage. It strains your innards. Tires you out. And it's likely to step up your menstrual flow. Leave the heavier chores to the huskier sex . . . you'll help *more* by keeping *healthy*.

Thumbs down on tennis—if you play it a la tournament. Tearing around a tennis court tempts nature to talk back. Like all "fierce fun" it should be postponed. (Unless your technique is the slow-motion type—with time out now and then).

(NO CAN DO)

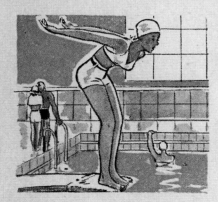

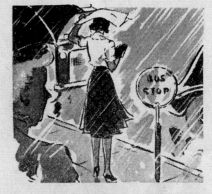

Hold it! Diving's not for you—for it's dollars to doughnuts the water's *cold*. And cold water shocks your system. You can bask on the beach and take the sun. (Go ahead. That's *good!*) But, unless it's fairly warm—lady beware the water.

Don't be a chill Jill! Chills usually cause trouble. Avoid getting wet feet ... catching cold. When you have a stormy-weather date, you needn't take a rain check if you wear rubbers, carry a bumbershoot. Otherwise, wait till the sun shines, Nellie!

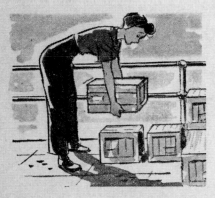

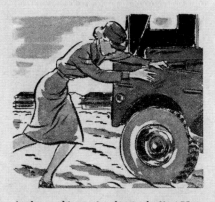

Why lift the dangerous way? There's a knack in avoiding strain. Bend knees. Keep your back straight, "tummy" in. Get close to the object—under, if possible. Lift upward, parallel with body. In carrying, divide weight evenly, or shift from left to right.

And put *this* on the don't-do list! You aren't built to cope with a balky car. Straining is harmful. *Now*, above all ... when it's apt to cause "floodings" ... innard injury. Observe this taboo at *home*, too. Don't wrestle with weighty furniture.

feet in ice water in order to stave off their periods before a big party. The way to rev the flow back up again? A hot tub and a cup of herbal tea was usually enough to do the trick.

But once Dr. Dixon got on a roll, he apparently couldn't stop theorizing, and those cold feet were just the tip of the iceberg. He wrote that girls from warm climates hit menarche earlier than those who grew up in chillier regions, who apparently only had their periods during the summer. He also expounded on the "artificial maturity" brought on by saucy novels, or too much time spent on art, music, or dancing. Any of these inherently unwholesome activities, he warned darkly, would most definitely cause puberty to start early.

Dr. Dixon wasn't alone in his nutball theories. In his 1898 book, *Confidential Talks with Young Women*, Dr. Lyman Sperry was right there wagging his finger reprovingly about those cold, wet feet of ours. He also put forth the idea that since the womb and nervous system were intricately connected, anger, grief, fear, anxiety, or depression could check one's flow. As a result, emotional girls should think twice before attending parties, picnics, or sleigh rides, all of which could stimulate a girl right into her own self-propelled menstrual suppression, wreaking havoc on her precious fertility. No smart-thinking girl should ever knowingly travel during the first few days of her period, as the stress and fatigue would throw off her schedule. But even if that dire event occurred, all she needed was a warm bed and a cup of hot tea, and everything would soon be as right as rain.

It wasn't just menstruation that Dr. Sperry had a bee in his bonnet about. A paid lecturer on "sanitary science"—the popular movement that extolled the importance of hygiene and railed against the terrifying, unseen world of germs—he had a virtual cow about masturbation, considered one of the great social evils of the time, as well as any indulgence in "lustful and lascivious thought." Sperry felt, perhaps a bit too feverishly, that girls hitting puberty needed to control their sexual urges, lest they permanently damage their reproductive organs. In fact, girls who "abused" those organs "seriously diminish not only their own capacity for happiness, but their power for producing healthy, happy children."

Professor T. W. Shannon, in his 1913 book *Self Knowledge and Guide to Sex Instruction*, was another nattering nabob of negativity when it came to the whole idea of female self-love. Girls who masturbated and poked around where they shouldn't be poking were clearly writing themselves a one-way ticket to lifelong pain, suffering, and worse. "The mind becomes sluggish and stupid," he thundered. "Memory fails and sometimes the poor victim becomes insane. This habit leads to a gloomy, despondent, discouraged state of mind. Because of this mental state, many commit suicide." At the same time, he urged mothers to teach their daughters that their reproductive organs were nothing to be ashamed of; instead, he wrote, they "form the sacred sanctuary which will one day enable her to become the sweetest and holiest of God's creatures—a pure, happy mother."

Is it hilariously campy or truly creepy to realize just how many outrageous, sometimes silly, often dangerous theories and myths have been dreamt up about menstruation—and how those far-fetched ideas still resonate in modern society?

Take a look at ads for menstrual suppression, menopause treatments, or medications for extreme PMS—they focus relentlessly on how much better a woman's life would be if only she could control her blood. So let's be frank: how far have we really come, when society is still pounding the message that our reproductive systems are faulty and need to be tinkered with, and that our bodies would work much, much better with a little help from the outside?

How did we get here? It's where we're headed that freaks us out.

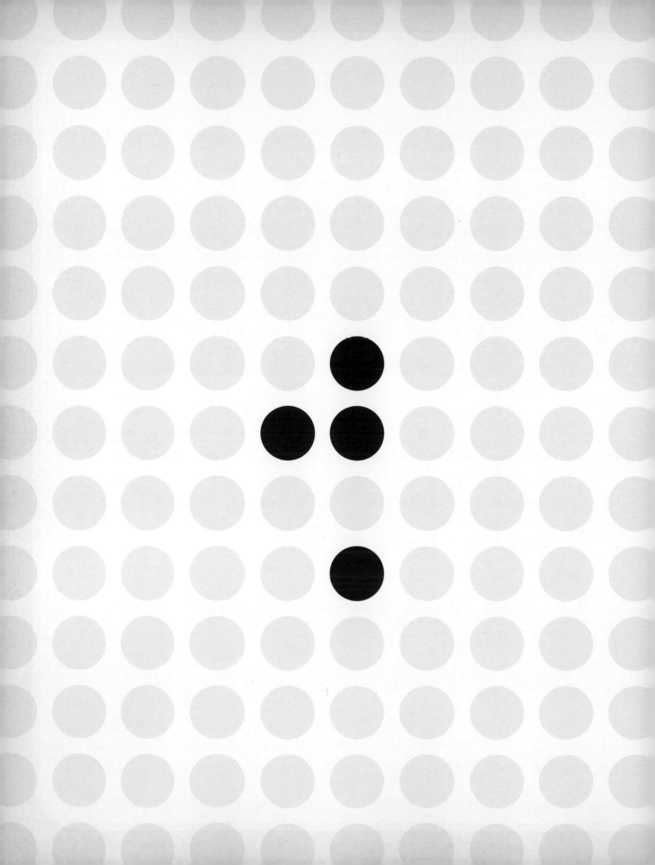

Chapter 4

HYSTERIA

ON A GENTEEL, TREE-LINED STREET NEAR OUR respective homes in New York City's Greenwich Village is a charming little shop exclusively dedicated to sex toys. Inside, cheerful, fresh-faced young men and women are happy to help customers ponder the options: a dominatrix catsuit made out of PVC, perhaps, or a titanium cock ring, multicolored condoms, pineapple-flavored lubricants, butt plugs. What catches our eye, however, is the extraordinary range of vibrators available: in various colors and sizes, rotating, waterproof, egg-shaped, filled with jelly. And we wonder: do any of the friendly, nipple-ringed staff realize that the vibrator's history is actually inextricably linked to the ancient story of hysteria and the uterus?

Hysteria, that mysterious catchall of female ailments that existed in recorded history for thousands of years, is a diagnosis that dates back to ancient Egypt. It's associated with out-of-control emotions, irrational fears, and unregulated, over-the-top behavior, but overwhelmingly, only in women. And believe it or not, one of the most popular treatments for hysteria that literally spanned centuries was manual stimulation to orgasm by a medical doctor.

Okay, it wasn't actually *called* an orgasm back then, it was a "hysterical paroxysm." And believe it or not, it wasn't even considered sexual; in a world ruled by a heterosexual, male-oriented notion of sex (i.e., vaginal intercourse in the missionary position), stimulating someone's clitoris was considered therapeutic and about as racy as bandaging a head wound. That being said, we find the whole thing more than a tad kinky. Just read the instructions Pieter van Forest wrote in 1653, which makes it all pretty clear to us: "A midwife should massage the genitalia with one finger inside, using oil of lilies, musk root, crocus or [something] similar. And in this way the afflicted woman can be aroused to a paroxysm."

Van Forest was far from the first to describe this method, and in such lingering detail, as an effective treatment for hysteria. Centuries earlier, Hippocrates, that father of modern medicine, mentioned a similar treatment in his writings. And Galen himself, that old second-century perv, wrote: "Following the warmth of the remedies and arising from the touch of the genital organs required by the treatment, there followed twitchings accompanied at the same time by pain and pleasure, after which she emitted turbid and abundant sperm. From that time on, she was free of all the evil she felt."

And yet, the medical profession emphatically did *not* suggest a woman try this at home by herself (perhaps with a nice glass of wine, listening to some music, and surrounded by cushions). No, it was a medical treatment to be provided by a professional—a doctor or midwife—at a scheduled appointment, for cold, hard cash. If one were lucky, one could even find someone to stop by for a house call.

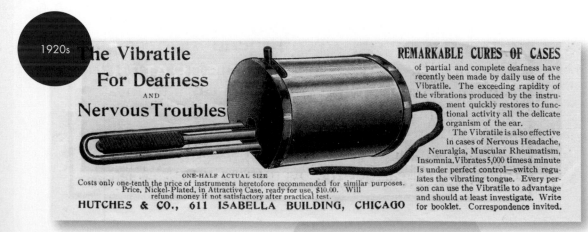

1920s

The Vibratile For Deafness AND Nervous Troubles

ONE-HALF ACTUAL SIZE

Costs only one-tenth the price of instruments heretofore recommended for similar purposes. Price, Nickel-Plated, in Attractive Case, ready for use, $10.00. Will refund money if not satisfactory after practical test.

HUTCHES & CO., 611 ISABELLA BUILDING, CHICAGO

REMARKABLE CURES OF CASES of partial and complete deafness have recently been made by daily use of the Vibratile. The exceeding rapidity of the vibrations produced by the instrument quickly restores to functional activity all the delicate organism of the ear.

The Vibratile is also effective in cases of Nervous Headache, Neuralgia, Muscular Rheumatism, Insomnia. Vibrates 5,000 times a minute Is under perfect control—switch regulates the vibrating tongue. Every person can use the Vibratile to advantage and should at least investigate. Write for booklet. Correspondence invited.

Going to the doctor's for such a treatment was nothing like putting on an oversize gown that ties in front and scooting your bare butt down to the end of the table where the stirrups are. Back then, a woman remained not only standing, but fully clothed; the doctor would have to bend down and reach up under all of her heavy draperies in order to locate the right spot, working completely by feel. Not surprisingly, the treatment was incredibly taxing; it probably took the hapless doctor time to even *find* the clitoris, and after that up to a full hour to achieve the desired result. Plus it was difficult; one doctor back in 1660 ruefully compared the technique to rubbing one's stomach with one hand while patting one's head with the other. As a result, midwives were often employed to do the actual handiwork.

But by the late nineteenth century, the second stage of the Industrial Revolution, which had already transformed farming, manufacturing, transportation, and the face of labor forever, also brought us the vibrator. Dr. J. M. Granville, a British physician, developed a mechanical model in 1883, and overnight, doctors found they could treat hysteria patients in mere minutes instead of hours.

What a boon! The vibrator quickly became a staple in doctors' offices, and as treatments sped up, revenue streams (ahem) shot through the roof. According to Rachel Maines in her 2001 book, *The Technology of Orgasm*, the eventual variety of vibrators offered in the late nineteenth century rivaled and possibly surpassed the inventory of today, even in the best-stocked sex shop: "musical vibrators, counterweighted vibrators, vibratory forks, undulating wire coils called vibratiles, vibrators that hung from the ceiling, vibrators attached to tables, floor models on rollers and portable devices . . . powered by electric current, battery, foot pedal, water turbine, gas engine or air pressure . . . at speeds ranging from 1,000 to 7,000 pulses per minute."

1920c

And with the first public utilities bringing electricity directly into the home, special vibrators were quickly developed and sold through catalogs for use in the privacy of one's own boudoir. The "electrotherapeutic industry" became wildly successful; vibrator ads began to jockey for dominance, discreetly, against ads for hair pomade, ribbons, and lavender soap in women's magazines like *Needle Craft, Modern Women*, and *Women's Home Companion*. One brand, the Moon Massage Vibrator, was advertised as "the little home doctor." Even the supremely square Sears Roebuck catalog carried, in a 1918 ad called "Aids That Every Woman Appreciates," a blurb for a portable vibrator that came with ominous-sounding attachments, like the "buffer" and "grinder." The vibrator was electrified nine years before the vacuum cleaner and beat electric frying pans by almost ten.

To say that there has always been an obvious need for genuine, clitoral-based sexual gratification for women—provided either by doctor, midwife, or mechanical/electrical device—seems to be quite the understatement. And yet, what's so odd about the need for female pleasure? Certainly, men have been availing themselves of the services of prostitutes from the moment those early hominids stood upright and certain women could say, "Hey there, sailor"; it's not called the world's oldest profession for nothing.

But what intrigues us is the fact that women's sexuality—both its repression and expression—has been perceived in such doggedly detached, clinical, and deliberately nonerotic terms, for thousands of years, whether consciously or unconsciously, as both the source of and solution to a concocted medical problem. Men have admittedly come up with some wacky notions before, but to us, this one really takes the cake.

So how did this all come about? And why?

And what *is* hysteria, anyway?

Hysteria was perhaps the greatest false diagnosis ever made in the history of Western medicine: a phony medical condition dating back to even before ancient Greece and only bowing out as an official disease when the American Psychiatric Association finally dropped the term in 1952. It included such an extraordinary range of symptoms, it's hard to imagine anyone reaching a diagnosis with a straight face. A partial list includes: nervousness, insomnia, faintness, chills, fluid retention, heaviness in the abdomen, depression, headache, upset stomach, loss of appetite, shortness of breath, irritability, unexplained laughter or crying, anxiety, a choking sensation, muscle spasms, convulsions, fatigue, loss of appetite, cold hands, cold feet, loss of sexual interest, heaving of the chest, a sudden throwing back of the head and body, "the tendency to cause trouble," and on, and on, and on, ad infinitum. Symptoms allegedly ran one Victorian doctor seventy-five pages in an unfinished list. And as one scans the seemingly bottomless inventory, one cannot help but notice the distinctly sexual nature of many of the symptoms: anxiety, sleeplessness, irritability, nervousness, erotic fantasy, sensations of heaviness in the abdomen, lower pelvic swelling, vaginal lubrication.

From the very beginning, hysteria was believed to be caused by the uterus and was even named after that pear-shaped pelvic pouch. And what we find especially telling is that the uterus, funnily enough, is *the only female organ for which there is no male counterpart.*

Think about it: men have breasts, the ovaries and testicles are both gonads, and one can go on and on throughout both male and female bodies, finding reasonable equivalents. But a male uterus? Nothing even comes close, unless one is generous and counts a beer belly. And thus due to its inherently and exclusively female essence, not to mention its seemingly magical ability to *make babies,* the innocent womb has since time immemorial been both whipping boy and Rorschach inkblot to men, the object of far too much masculine speculation and fantasy, as well as the brunt of their frequently cruel medical attentions.

In an ancient Egyptian papyrus from around 1900 B.C. (one of the earliest records in medical history, we'd like to point out), aberrant behavior in women was already being commented on and the theory put forth that a wandering uterus was the root of their problems. As a result, Egyptian doctors routinely fed noxious substances to their female patients, hoping to drive the uterus away from the lungs and throat. Alternately, they placed sweet-smelling substances on the vulva, trying to coax it back into place. The ancient Greeks (who otherwise made huge strides in medical knowledge and conceivably should have known better) agreed wholeheartedly that the uterus was in fact rampaging through the body, in a frantic search for babies.

And so what was the cure for a cranky womb? The Greeks decided that the only way to both cheer it up and promptly relieve the symptoms of hysteria was marriage—or to put it more bluntly, lots and lots of sex. Marital relations would satisfy the uterus's need for moisture (from semen, if we need to draw you a picture), as well as give it those babies it was seeking so desperately.

Prescribing marital sex for hysteria was popular until the Middle Ages, when fundamentalist religious fervor replaced rational thought. Not that using sex to placate an angry organ was exactly what one would normally call rational; yet it was better than the Catholic Church's position on hysteria, which was that it was caused by possession by evil spirits.

During the Middle Ages, which lasted from the fifth century to the sixteenth, things previously taken for granted, like science, medicine, democracy, and philosophy, were flung out the window like so much offal as the Church tightened its already mighty grip on society itself. Any undiagnosable illnesses or instances of bizarre behavior were now diagnosed, conveniently if not constructively, as having been brought on by the devil himself. So instead of being summarily married off, women unfortunate enough to merit the diagnosis of hysteria were instead tried in Church courts and often prosecuted as witches.

To be honest, the Church during the Middle Ages seemed to be particularly down on all women, and not just hysterical ones. Midwives in particular seemed to merit an especially hairy eyeball, what with all that spooky healing knowledge, those eerily effective herbal remedies, and that life-saving familiarity with childbirth, contraception, and other gynecological matters. Clearly in league with You-Know-Who, they too were frequently prosecuted by the Church as witches.

Fortunately, there were still intrepid individuals who bucked the oppressive religious trend and furtively continued to explore science. Not swallowing the idea that demonic possession was responsible for any kind of pathology, these men began once again to question how the body actually worked, theorizing about its many systems.

It's important to keep in mind that throughout virtually all of history, even in supposedly enlightened times, a woman's body and mind were considered significantly inferior to and less evolved than a man's: designed for bearing children, but still weaker, feebler, and more poorly made. An 1848 obstetrics text wrote that "she (woman) has a head almost too small for intellect, but just big enough for love." What's more, her body was a total mystery, as well, both intimidating and scary: periodically bleeding, producing children, and so on. Until the 1700s, female genitalia was considered to be all lumped together, without distinct vocabulary to distinguish its different parts.

In the nineteenth century, however, Jean-Martin Charcot, one of the earliest modern neurologists, put forth the first scientific argument against the centuries-old wandering-womb theory and suggested that hysteria was instead a brain-based phenomenon, with physical manifestations. Two of his students, Pierre Janet and Sigmund Freud, went on to posit that hysteria was psychological in origin, with symptoms arising from the subconscious. In other words, unresolved conflict manifested itself symbolically as physical symptoms. This theory was a huge step forward in many ways, as well as a disturbing step back.

Freud himself, who once wrote that "women oppose change, receive passively, and add nothing of their own," clearly had issues of his own when it came to unresolved conflict, especially with regard to women. He freely projected his own sexual insecurities while attributing possible causes of hysteria: he suggested penis envy, the Oedipal complex, and castration anxiety, all of which indicate, to us at least, a certain infantile phallocentrism. But he ultimately came closest to the mark when he concluded that hysteria represented unresolved sexual conflict. To his mind, many women, if not most, were sexually frigid.

These weren't quite the fightin' words then that they are now. The Victorian era was almost cartoonishly repressed and repressive, especially for middle- and upper-class women, and it was the rare female who could actually get jiggy in the bedroom. The ideal woman of Freud's day was passive, modest, restricted with heavy clothing, and uninterested in sex. In fact, hygiene manuals actually warned against "spasmodic convulsion" in the woman during sex, lest it interfere with all-important conception. With that as the wifely role model, is it any surprise that prostitution became such a boom business during the Victorian era?

Perhaps not coincidentally, hysteria experienced its heyday in the mid- to late nineteenth century, sweeping through the middle and upper-middle echelons of British and American society like a forest fire run amok, afflicting an untold number of women. In 1871, women's rights educator Catherine Beecher wrote despairingly of "hopeless invalidism," "the mysterious epidemic," and "a terrible decay of female health all over the land, which was increasing in a most alarming ratio." Wealthy women took to the supine position in record numbers, and as a direct result, a morbid sickliness became *le dernier cri*, the latest romanticized aesthetic ideal. Artists and poets lovingly described pasty, tremblingly frail women languishing on their chaises, smelling salts in hand. Ghastly white pallor was also deemed a fashion "do," as it bespoke the refinement of one who didn't labor in the fields (a robust tan being a definite fashion "don't"). To achieve this rarefied, Bozo the Clown look, women routinely painted their skin with white lead, zinc oxide, mercury, lead, or nitrate of silver . . . which led to other, far more serious medical problems.

Speaking of fashion, it was the hellishly restrictive clothing styles of the day that also created severe health problems, many of which would have certainly contributed to a diagnosis of hysteria. As Barbara Ehrenreich and Deirdre English noted in their 1989 book, *For Her Own Good*: "Corsets exerted, on the average, 21 pounds of pressure on a woman's organs, and extremes up to 88 pounds had been measured. . . . Some of the results of tight lacing were shortness of breath, constipation, weakness, indigestion. Among the long-term effects were bent or broken ribs, displacement of the liver, uterine prolapse. In some cases the uterus would be gradually forced by the pressure of the corset down through the vagina."

Another possible cause of hysteria was dietary—namely too much sugar enjoyed by middle- and upper-class women, which led not only to tooth decay, but also infections, digestive problems, and low energy. In 1898, Dr. Lyman Sperry, the author of *Confidential Talks with Young Women*, blamed excessive sweet eating as the undiagnosed cause of many mental and physical problems of the day.

To be fair, not everyone bought into the whole idea of hysteria; in fact, many skeptics believed women were fabricating such attacks in a Victorian manifestation

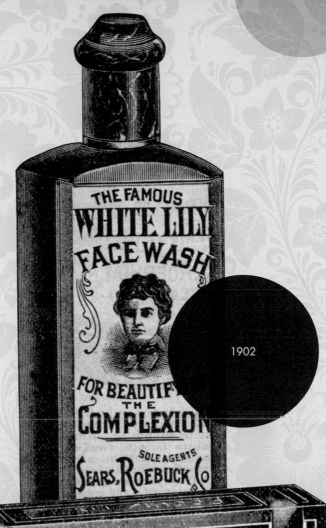

THE FAMOUS
WHITE LILY
FACE WASH

FOR BEAUTIFY
THE
COMPLEXION

SOLE AGENTS
SEARS, ROEBUCK Co

1902

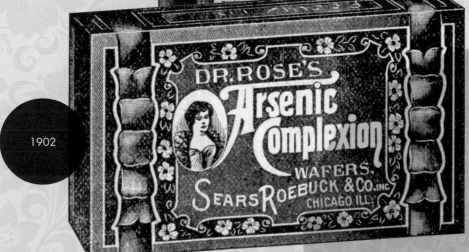

DR. ROSE'S
Arsenic
Complexion
WAFERS.
Sears Roebuck & Co. INC
CHICAGO ILL.

1902

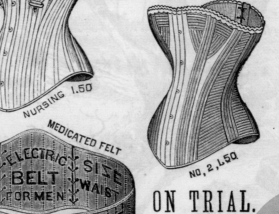
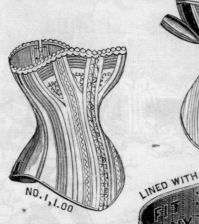
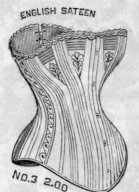
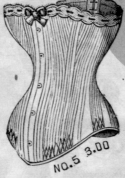

of the Drama Queen just to get attention. Several pointed out that hysterics never had fits when they were alone. Plus, the mysterious ailment only seemed to affect the women who could actually afford to be terminally bedridden; you sure didn't catch the working class falling prey to hysteria. To deal with an outburst, doctors suggested suffocating the woman until her fits stopped, or beating her with a wet towel or otherwise humiliating her in front of family and friends until she finally quit.

Supporters retorted that physical frailty went with an innately superior refinement and sensitivity. But whatever the reason, it was invariably wealthier women, with too much time on their hands and too little to do, who sank in record numbers into chronically debilitating conditions such as hysteria, nervous depression, melancholia, and neurasthenia.

As a result, all sorts of innovative (i.e., horrifyingly sadistic) therapies were explored for the treatment of hysteria: heat, X-rays, bleaching, injections, electrical shocks. Doctors experimented with sticking leeches on the vulva, cauterizing the cervix, or even surgically removing the clitoris.

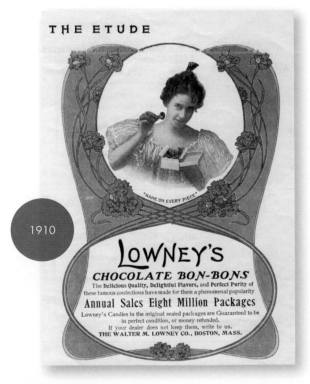

THE ETUDE

NAME ON EVERY PIECE

LOWNEY'S
CHOCOLATE BON-BONS
The Delicious Quality, Delightful Flavors, and Perfect Purity of these famous confections have made for them a phenomenal popularity
Annual Sales Eight Million Packages
Lowney's Candies in the original sealed packages are Guaranteed to be in perfect condition, or money refunded.
If your dealer does not keep them, write to us.
THE WALTER M. LOWNEY CO., BOSTON, MASS.

1910

Funnily enough, none of these or other such treatments seemed to work. This included hysterectomy or ovariotomy (removal of the ovaries), a procedure that was first performed in Greece back in 120 B.C. and came roaring back into popularity at the height of the hysteria epidemic. Despite the 50 percent death rate, it was recommended not only for hysteria, but also for masturbation, uncomfortable menstruation, even too much libido. Patients were usually brought in by their husbands, and without a second thought doctors ripped out their healthy reproductive organs, striving for placid, postsurgical women in a sort of bizarre reproductive spin on the lobotomy.

Grim times, no? And so, this leads us back, finally, not only to Freud, but Hippocrates, Galen, and the rest of that ancient gang.

Masturbation was viewed as something unwholesome and unnatural, while therapeutic stimulation was simply a means to an end, namely to relieve hysteria.

Could it be that they actually had a point? Was it really sex, or rather, the lack of sex, *good* sex, and the accompanying buildup of frustration that caused the thing called hysteria in the first place? Certainly, if it had been untold millions of men rather than women who routinely went without sexual release for years, we would have imagined not only hysteria but perhaps actual nuclear Armageddon to have erupted long ago. Whatever the actual problem, remedies such as those from ancient Greece once again became the go-to answer for female malaise.

Consider the so-called water cure, popularized by Austrian physicist Vicenz Priessnitz and perhaps the biggest health fad of the mid-nineteenth century, lasting well until the 1920s. One may immediately conjure up quaint, sepia-tinted images of women cavorting in the cold surf in checked mob caps, stockings to the knee, and frilly bathing costumes, taking in the wholesome salt air. In fact, the cure consisted of high-powered water douches that were aimed squarely at the genital area for the express purpose of inducing orgasm.

The water cure was an instant hit, and not just for the obvious reasons. At the time, having a hysterectomy was like playing Russian roulette with a loaded gun; it was a relief to have a medical procedure that entailed little risk other than getting one's hair wet. And did it work? Consider R. J. Lane, who, when writing about a British spa in 1851, described the effects of the water cure thusly: "Persons are frequently known, on coming out of the douche, to declare that they feel as much elation and buoyancy of spirits, as if they had been drinking champagne." Warm water or cold was sprayed from hoses hung high above or while patients were seated in tubs with jets pumping underneath. Water cures were soon all the rage, combining unprecedented sexual satisfaction with a wholesome-sounding vacation. Soon, women wanted more sessions, and then more, and more; one therapist said he had "difficulty in keeping them within rational limits."

And how much of a surprise was that? In the nineteenth and early twentieth centuries, it was apparently both socially acceptable and medically approved for women to experience orgasm, but only in a controlled, deliberately nonsexual manner: in a doctor's office, at a Saratoga Springs douching room, via a doctor-prescribed horseback ride or train trip over bumpy tracks (we're not making this stuff up), or using a jolting chair or electrified rocking chair specifically invented for this purpose. Appointments were made, money changed hands, and sexual release was effected dutifully, as a form of therapy. Yet at the same time, masturbation remained strictly verboten.

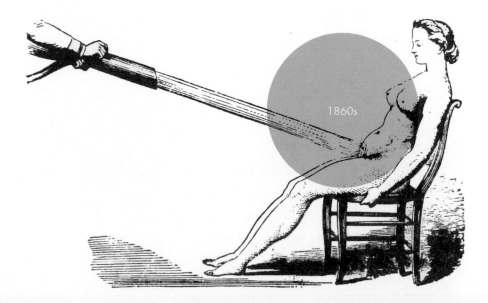

Masturbation was not only a one-way ticket to hell, it was addictive and physically dangerous, as well. In his 1898 book, *Confidential Talks with Young Women*, Dr. Lyman Sperry didn't mince words: "Every part of the body is abused and injured by it. You need not think it harmless at first because you do not feel those effects at first, for they come on so slowly that children are very often near death before they or their friends find out what is the matter with them; and if they do not die, the evil will cling to them and make them miserable through all their lives." He also darkly insinuated that masturbators would swiftly become either insane or mentally retarded, and would very likely commit suicide.

This may all seem like a hopeless contradiction, and yet it makes a certain perverse sense. Western society has always assumed that women experience pleasure exclusively via the vagina, i.e., from intercourse with a man. Only vaginal penetration was considered stimulating to women, which is why the speculum and tampon were so controversial when they were introduced and the vibrator basically given a free pass. As a result, masturbation was viewed as something unwholesome and unnatural, while therapeutic stimulation was simply a means to an end, namely to relieve hysteria.

Even though hysteria was finally disavowed by the American Psychiatric Association in the early 1950s, the notion lingered on—now thought to be a result of a woman's frigidity. Subtly, the prevailing attitude had shifted: the woman was no longer the passive victim of hysteria due to her uterus, but was instead somehow at fault due

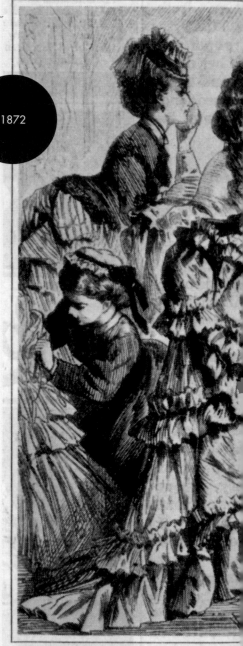

DRAWN BY J. N. HYDE.   FRANK LESLIE'S ILLUSTRATED

Scen

1872

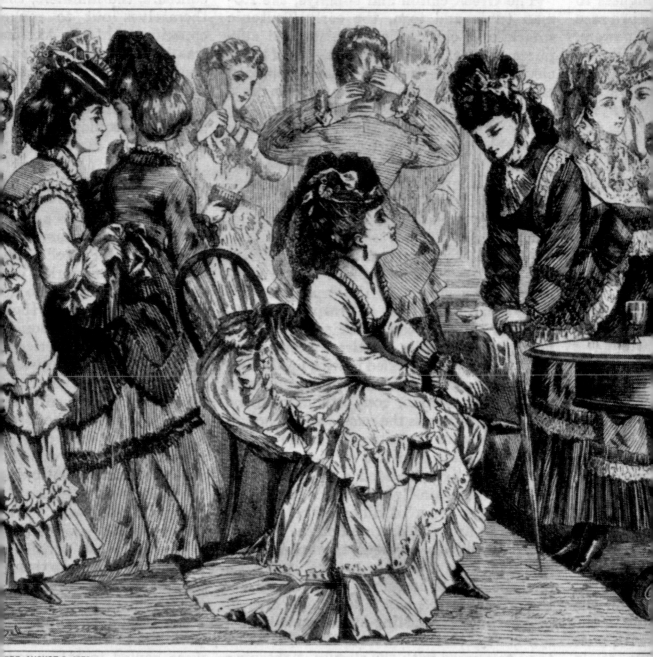

PER, AUGUST 3, 1872

the Ladies' Parlor of the Grand Union Hotel, Saratoga, 1872

Frank Leslie's Illustrated Newspaper

to her innate coldness and lack of interest in sex. From the 1954 *Illustrated Encyclopedia of Sex:* "There are women who have 'grown cold,' women who, as a result of the deadly monotony of their marriage, have gradually lost their former undoubted potency and sometimes even their sexual desire. In such cases the medical man can do nothing. These emotionally dead people should be left to their dead, and our efforts should be devoted to the countless other unfortunate people whom it is still possible to help."

There are dozens of conflicting explanations and theories explaining what hysteria was, what caused it and cured it, and even reasons for its great epidemic in the late nineteenth century. While many blamed frigidity, others blamed the physical constraints of fashion, the effects of diet, the need for children. Wherever the truth actually lies, we do feel that lying beneath the bogus, catchall unspecificity of the diagnosis, *something was actually going on . . .* something that brought genuine suffering to untold numbers of women. The question is, what was it exactly? And perhaps just as significantly, what brought it on?

We're pretty sure that regular lack of sexual fulfillment may well have contributed to the unhappiness many women clearly felt for so many thousands of years. Yet can we get both political and conspiracy theorish for a moment?

Could what was historically called hysteria—widespread instances of clinical depression, unhappiness, anxiety, anger—have been a simple product not so much of sexual or maternal frustration, but of actual systematized oppression? After all, throughout history, women had no rights or autonomy, and were routinely barred from higher education, property ownership, the right to vote, careers. Could it be that when anyone is faced with such fundamental obstacles to happiness and self-actualization, even a whiz-bang orgasm isn't enough to make things all better again?

By the mid-nineteenth century, change was in the air. The suffrage movement was on the rise, and women were fighting for higher education, as well. The possibilities were tantalizing, and yet the pressures brought by such change were enormous, taking their toll on women both mentally and emotionally. Margaret Sanger, the great birth control crusader, spent time incapacitated by deep depression. Jane Addams, social activist and the first American woman to be awarded the Nobel Peace Prize, was also debilitated by depression for seven years. And Alice James, brilliant sister of novelist Henry and philosopher William, was chronically beset by nervous breakdowns that ruined her life.

Charlotte Perkins Gilman, an early feminist writer, was diagnosed with hysteria in the late 1800s and was sent to Dr. Silas Weir Mitchell, a hysteria specialist. He famously offered depressed men the "West Cure," in which he urged them to go west, have rugged adventures in the wild, and then sit down and write about it. To his female patients, however, he prescribed the "Rest Cure"—which consisted of isolated bed rest for as long as two months, forced feedings, occasional electroshock therapy, and absolutely no reading and writing. Gilman later wrote damningly of her ordeal in her terrifying story, published in 1892, *The Yellow Wallpaper*, in which the heroine is literally driven insane by such a cure.

It wasn't until the frighteningly recent 1950s that the diagnosis of hysteria, at least as it related to unexplainable female behavior, was finally, at long last, laid to rest, after one of the longest runs by any faux medical condition in history. By then, the field of psychology had far greater understanding about depression, anxiety, and other mood disorders, and so women suffering from any of those could now get a more concrete diagnosis than hysteria, as well as a more appropriate therapy. What's more, by the 1950s, women had vastly more opportunities to be engaged in the world around them and challenged by their lives, strength, and interests. The 1950s may not have been a feminist mecca, but women had far more rights than ever before in history.

But here's an interesting thought: hysteria, which was one of the most frequently diagnosed diseases in history, was officially removed from their *Diagnostic and Statistical Manual* by the American Psychiatric Association in 1952. And yet the following year, the term "premenstrual syndrome" was coined by Dr. Katharina Dalton. The National Health Service currently lists over 150 symptoms for PMS, including: feeling irritable and bad tempered, fluid retention and feeling bloated, mood swings, feeling upset or emotional, insomnia (trouble sleeping), difficulty concentrating, backache, muscle and joint pain, breast tenderness, tiredness, appetite changes, or food cravings.

Sound familiar? Hysteria by any other name . . .

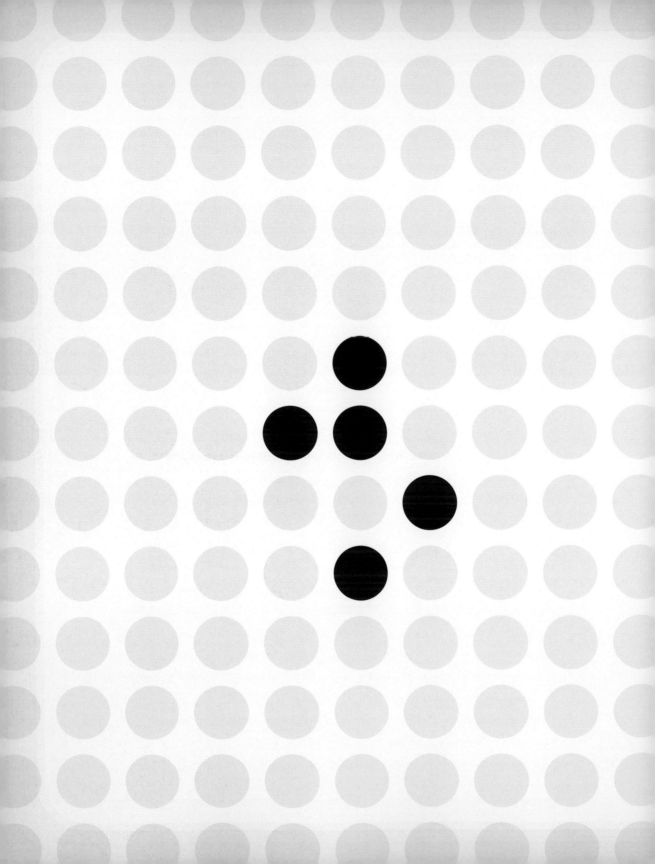

Chapter 5

SEEING RED

ARRIDAN. SHREW. BATTLEAXE, SPITFIRE, NAG.
Termagant, if you're feeling literary, or just plain bitch, if you're not.

There have been derogatory words for moody, temperamental, argumentative women for centuries. When Shakespeare wrote *The Taming of the Shrew*, after all, he sure wasn't talking about how to train a small foraging land mammal. The word "bitch" goes back to at least 1400. In an 1811 British dictionary, it's described as "the most offensive appellation that can be given to an English woman, even more provoking than that of 'whore.'"

While one may ponder at length about which is actually worse, being called a bitch or a whore, the fact remains that society seems to hold the Difficult Woman in a truly special position of distaste and contempt, even hatred. While no one really enjoys being shrieked at by anyone, regardless of the shrieker's gender, there appears to be far greater dislike of the woman, rather than the man, who blows up, chokes with quivering fury, or sobs with impotent despair.

And we're not just talking about men who hate it. Women are often the first to accuse another woman of being a bitch, and they often secretly find endless blame and deep humiliation when it comes to their own frayed tempers, angry outbursts, and

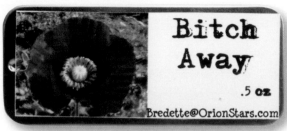

© 2008 Bredette Dyer, www.orionstars.com

tearful tirades. We ourselves have lain awake at three in the morning, bitterly regretting the way we had screamed at our families earlier, burst into racking sobs at a difficult meeting, blown up at a well-intentioned spouse. We picture our faces red with anger, our eyes bulging with rage and/or self-pitying tears, and we feel a deep, quivering shame. *Why did I do that? Why didn't I just let it go? What's wrong with me, anyway?*

After all, you'd have to be either Madonna or just weirdly, preternaturally self-assured not to have internalized the overriding message that's still being fed to every woman around the world and throughout history, since birth: that the truly feminine female is the one who is boundlessly patient, as well as impossibly sympathetic, eternally sweet-tempered, and just plain good (whatever the hell that means). While men have pretty much, since time immemorial, been the ones responsible for 99 percent of all violent crimes and 99.9 percent of all wars, it is still the woman who loses her temper who seems to trigger the greatest alarm and harshest condemnation from one and all.

Why is this? We understand that we, the fairer sex, may not be brimming over with even one-fifth as much chest-thumping testosterone as are the guys, but still, we're only human, aren't we? We don't see men being castigated for their outbursts of anger or their fits of depression, nor do we find many of them losing much sleep about it, either. Anger and despair may not necessarily be the most entrancing of emotions, it's true, but occasionally, they're the only appropriate responses to a bad situation—i.e., anything difficult that happens to us when we don't have enough hours in the day, or money, or help, or sleep.

When it comes to women, obviously, you can't talk about anger, anxiety, and depression without also mentioning the 800-pound gorilla in the room. We're talking about the extra factor that may very well play a mysterious if complex part in our occasionally ungovernable emotions . . . and that, of course, is PMS.

FEMCARE WEIGHS IN ON MOOD SWINGS

Blues sometimes come right before your period. But they don't always have to come. Some girls expect them . . . make a habit of them. Smart girls won't give in to them. They take their minds off themselves . . . do things they enjoy doing—like dancing, listening to records. They find that doing happy things helps them feel happy—look happy. **—TAMPAX (1966)**

Many women imagine they feel worse than they actually do. They get in a dither, or down in the dumps, just by thinking too much about themselves.

—KOTEX (1943)

Mental attitudes frequently affect bodily functions. Fretting, worry, self-pity can make a person sick and miserable when there is no physical reason for being either. If we dramatize little discomforts . . . if we think of menstruation as being "sick" or as the "curse" . . . we only make it unpleasant for ourselves.

—BELTX (1955)

It's no coincidence that mothers who complain about menstrual pain have daughters who develop pains, too.

—MODESS (1954)

A poor mental attitude will do much towards tensing muscles and causing cramps. **—TAMPAX (1966)**

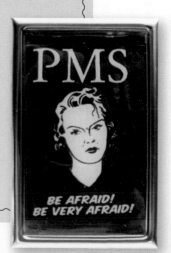

So what is PMS, exactly?

Premenstrual syndrome is defined as a collection of physical and emotional symptoms that appear in the week before one's period and disappear shortly after flow begins. If you're American, you probably think *all* women suffer from PMS, that it's an inevitable monthly madness that overtakes any female of reproductive age, an inescapable nightmare of bloated bellies, torrents of tears, and snapping tempers. And if you think this, there's at least one good reason why you do: premenstrual syndrome, not unlike its elderly grandmother, hysteria, has been defined and redefined by numerous experts over the years to the point where it's a bulging grab bag of symptoms, both physical and emotional, that can afflict, to varying degrees, practically any woman possessing a menstrual cycle. These symptoms, some contradictory, can include not only bloating, headaches, cramps, swollen feet, tender breasts, acne, nausea, weight gain, and fatigue, but also depression, insomnia, sleeplessness, lethargy, anxiety, anger, social withdrawal, difficulty thinking, and (how's this for a symptom?) a craving for carbohydrates. Since it was first classified, PMS has come to boast more than 150 identified symptoms.

This, to our jaundiced eye, is what we would call throwing the net a tad wide. It's no wonder women are absolutely convinced they suffer from PMS. With so many symptoms and such broad and fuzzy definitions, we're surprised to find it doesn't also apply to men, the elderly, and household pets, as well. And yet get this: there is virtually no consensus among the many, many "experts" on the subject as to what exactly causes PMS, how to treat it . . . or even what it is.

The heightened emotions and various physical symptoms many women experience in the week before their period were first identified in 1931 by Dr. Robert Frank, who called it "premenstrual tension." Previously, women who complained about it to their doctors were bluntly labeled "neurotic," "nervous," or "hysterical" and summarily sent on their not-so-merry way. The term "premenstrual syndrome," or PMS, was coined by British physician Dr. Katharina Dalton in 1953, who continued until her death in 2004 to be a veritable guru on the subject, gradually creating a mighty kingdom of bestselling books, court appearances as an expert witness, speaking engagements, and the first-ever PMS clinic from it.

The real glory days of PMS occurred in the early 1980s, when it seemed that every single women's magazine boasted a cover story about it, and any bookstore worth its salt stocked literally dozens of self-help titles telling women how to deal with it. Picking up where the outdated diagnosis of hysteria had left off, PMS became the universal female syndrome accepted by doctors, scientists, and laypeople everywhere, an inarguable fact of life for most, if not all, women.

And yet, how common is PMS, anyway? This is by no means a simple question with a black-and-white answer, because there's very little consensus among experts, doctors, scholars, researchers, even women themselves. In fact, studies on PMS to date have varied so wildly in their findings, the ensuing data is practically pointless. With so many possible symptoms, it turns out you could convincingly argue that anywhere from 5 percent to 97 percent of all women suffer from it at some time in their lives. Real useful, huh?

What's more, there have been disconcerting studies that link PMS and mental health. Most women who go to PMS clinics, for example, already suffer from preexisting depression. According to *The New Our Bodies, Ourselves*, PMS sufferers tend to have lower self-esteem than those who aren't afflicted, and are likelier to feel more out of control of their lives and guiltier about losing their tempers. A 1985 study showed that about two-thirds of women with a history of major affective disorder (such as depression) also suffer badly from PMS. If you flip that equation around, it turns out that most women with severe PMS have some preexisting history of depression and/or anxiety disorder, as well.

PMS symptoms appear to be at their worst when a woman is approximately thirty-five; in fact, a 1963 study even referred to premenstrual moodiness as "mid-thirties syndrome." One possible reason comes from a 1980 study, which finds that whereas fewer women in their twenties and forties ovulate in every cycle, nearly 92 percent of women in their thirties do. Does this mean PMS is somehow linked to ovulation? We're sorry to have to report this, but the scientific response is: who the hell knows?

Another explanation might be that most women who report severe PMS are mothers of young children. If PMS is in fact linked to stress, the mid-thirties can certainly be said to be an especially stressful time. In a recent study, almost half of PMS sufferers also reported marriage problems. More provocatively, a study recently suggested women who complain the most about PMS also tend to be more socially conservative, strongly endorsing a traditional female role as homemaker and mother.

So what are we to make of this hodgepodge of theories and conjecture?

Much of it seems to imply that PMS is purely psychological . . . when we all know that's not true. Our monthly emotional roller-coaster ride, bloating, and insomnia are not only real, but they're a purely physical problem based on our womanly hormones.

Or are they?

SYMPTOMS OF PMS . . . OR OF BEING HUMAN?

Abdominal cramps, absentmindedness, acne, aggressiveness, alcohol intolerance, angry outbursts, anxiety, argumentativeness, asthma, back pain, balance problems, being accident-prone, breast swelling and pain, compulsive eating, confusion, constipation, cravings for salty or sweet foods, crying jags, decreased energy, depression, diarrhea, difficulty concentrating, dizziness, edema (visible swelling, particularly in the hands, feet, and legs), edginess, energy bursts, fainting, fatigue, feeling out of control, food binges, fuzzy thinking, greasy hair, headaches, heart palpitations, hives, hopelessness, indecision, insomnia, irritability, judgment lapses, lack of coordination, lethargy, libido changes, loneliness, lowered self-esteem, migraines, mood swings, muscle aches, nausea, overeating, panic attacks, pelvic cramps, sadness, sinus problems, sore throat, tearfulness, tension, urinary problems, weight gain.

Actually—and you'll have to hold on to your hats for this one—contrary to popular wisdom and all those time-worn complaints about our raging hormones, *there is no real evidence of a hormonal basis for PMS.*

Did that sink in yet? We're frankly still processing it ourselves. And this isn't some kind of crazy conspiracy theory being pushed by either hard-core feminists or woman-hating reactionaries; this is hard, scientific fact. In other words, women who claim to suffer from PMS and women who don't have literally identical hormonal cycles.

What's more, there is absolutely no diagnostic test in the world that can conclusively determine whether or not a woman actually has PMS: no blood test, no monitor, no scientific way to detect traces of crazy-making chemicals lurking in our saliva or hair follicles or whatever. There is some evidence, given the prevalence of PMS among twins, that there may be a genetic component . . . but what that is is anyone's guess. Currently, researchers have been focusing on the possible effect of sex hormones on central nervous system neurotransmitters. Nevertheless, when it comes to concrete theories about what actually causes PMS, it appears as if researchers are still spitting in the air.

Not surprisingly, due to such incredibly fuzzy boundaries, PMS tends to be self-reported or, more spookily, reported by one's partner or colleagues. There are upward of 115 "PMS clinics" around the country; at those clinics, as well as in online groups, women are frequently urged to self-diagnose. Yet how can a woman really say if she has PMS when even the experts can't agree on what it is?

At the very least, a formal evaluation of PMS includes a thorough physical and gynecological exam, as well as a psychiatric assessment and medical history. Further psychological and lab testing may be done, as well. Even so, PMS is only officially diagnosed when a doctor can then confirm a pattern of symptoms that occur in the five days before the period for at least three cycles in a row; that the symptoms end within four days after the period stops; and, perhaps most crucially, *that the symptoms interfere with at least some aspects of the woman's normal life.*

That being said, other conditions can be and frequently are mistaken for PMS. Clinical depression and anxiety disorders, not surprisingly, are often confused with

PMS, because many of their symptoms are, well, *kinda sorta exactly the same.* To make things even more bewildering, conditions like manic depression and anxiety disorders often get worse during the premenstrual time; an otherwise dormant mental problem can suddenly flourish, as well. (In fact, one theory suggests that the word "lunatic" came about when it was observed that mental crises tended to follow the lunar/menstrual cycle of twenty-eight days.) So who the heck knows what's actually going on with that monthly tantrum of yours?

What's more, women who are entering menopause can also experience PMS-esque symptoms, like fatigue and mood swings. This is pretty normal, but there are also serious medical conditions that can eerily resemble PMS, problems you definitely wouldn't want to mess around with. These include irritable bowel syndrome, lupus, and chronic fatigue syndrome, as well as endocrine and thyroid problems—all of which can regularly flare up in the premenstrual time.

But don't get us wrong, here.

Just because PMS is clearly a strangely blurry, hard-to-define occurrence doesn't mean that unpleasant premenstrual symptoms are just in a woman's head. Mood swings, painful breasts, and fatigue before one's period are definitely real, a monthly physiological fact of life for many, if not most, women. And despite being one of the most wildly over- and misdiagnosed conditions in the Western world, PMS is still a genuine problem for millions. According to the American College of Obstetricians and Gynecologists, something like 85 percent of all women suffer from at least one of the typical symptoms, to varying degrees.

We ourselves have yet to meet a girl or woman who didn't sprout at least one pimple, gorge out on at least one pan of brownies, or feel truly, utterly convinced that she didn't have any real friends in the world the week before her period. The fact is, certain cyclical fluctuations in mood and the monthly reappearance of certain physical symptoms are clearly totally normal for most, if not all, healthy women of reproductive age. *Only when the premenstrual symptoms become such a problem that they significantly interfere with our normal lives can a woman really be said to suffer from PMS.*

For a small percentage, the premenstrual time looms as a monthly menace, one fraught with genuine concern. When a woman finds herself truly debilitated by not only horrible physical symptoms, but psycho mood swings, the kind that every month threaten to leave her home, work, and all relationships around her in smoldering ashes, she is said to suffer from Premenstrual Dysphoric Disorder, or PMDD.

PMDD is the super-duper, bad-ass-mother version of PMS that is said to affect anywhere from 3 to 8 percent of all women. Symptoms generally kick in from one to two weeks before flow starts, and subside several days after. For women who suffer from PMDD, this can therefore mean more than *half of each month* is spent feeling like Snow White's evil stepmother, smoking crack, on steroids.

For years, the supposed gold standard for treating PMDD was the hormone progesterone. This idea was touted by Dr. Katharina Dalton, the person who coined the term in the first place, and was much ballyhooed in her 1978 bestseller, *Once a Month,* and in PMS clinics around the country. Yet not only did critics point out attractive side effects such as depression, swelling, bleeding, and possibly increased rates of cancer, it turned out progesterone worked no better than placebos and was basically snake oil with a pedigree.

Since 2001, the single most popular way to treat women who suffer from PMDD has been a prescription drug called Sarafem (aka fluoxetine), first manufactured by Eli Lilly and Company, and now by Warner Chilcott. Sarafem (a drug whose name is clearly meant to evoke the "seraphim," the highest-ranked, most divine form of angel in the Christian celestial pecking order and something we should obviously be aspiring to be each month) is an antidepressant from the selective serotonin reuptake inhibitor class, a chemical twin to Prozac.

Do you remember Prozac? Sure you do. If you're old enough to wax fondly about the 1990s, you probably remember the insanely successful, green-and-white antidepressant manufactured by Eli Lilly, the one that spawned all those books and magazine articles and jokes on late-night television. Prozac went along its wildly profitable way until 2001, when the patent expired and fluoxetine went generic. Prices for the capsule immediately plummeted by about 80 percent.

Yet by then, the FDA had already quietly approved Sarafem. Sarafem costs three and a half times more than Prozac, even though it still has the exact same active ingredient, only now presented in girlish shades of yellow (and previously pink and lavender) rather than androgynous green and white. And if you're wondering darkly if the FDA knows about any of this, keep in mind that this is pharmaceutical business as usual.

What makes this especially galling is that while fluoxetine is now available generically for three and a half times less than Sarafem, doctors were forbidden for years to substitute the generic when writing a prescription to treat PMDD. This is because the FDA "Orange Book," which routinely lists drugs and their generic equivalents, claimed that Sarafem has no generic, because Warner Chilcott is the exclusive patent holder. Sarafem capsules only became available as a generic in May 2008.

Wild, no?

And so, back to the underlying question: what *are* PMS and PMDD, exactly? And how are we supposed to deal with them?

Most women clearly do have emotional and physical symptoms in the week before their period. And while we hate to be the ones who say it, since the condition itself is so poorly understood, there doesn't appear to be a single panacea or magic bullet that can handle them. Some studies show that regular exercise reduces anxiety; and many women we know swear by cutting down on salt, sugar, and caffeine, taking diuretics, and practicing stress-reduction techniques like yoga and meditation. Therapy or even talking about your symptoms to female friends can be a help, as well. We ourselves find that taking daily calcium and vitamin E supplements seems to help markedly with both the Cruella De Vil–esque temper swings and breast tenderness. Unfortunately, very few studies of these treatments have involved double-blind evaluations that would truly prove just what's effective and what isn't.

It's worth keeping another tidbit in mind. Even the underlying assumption that conditions like PMS and PMDD actually exist is by no means universal, even though both are widely accepted as medical fact across the United States. Many countries have never heard of either; while it's accepted worldwide that most women are indeed affected by their premenstrual cycles, the bloating, tears, and temper that seem to freak

Americans out so much don't seem to be viewed in such a negative, pathologized way elsewhere. In 1987, medical anthropologist Thomas Johns made the point that even though premenstrual symptoms have long been universally recognized, PMS only appears in Western industrial cultures, and then only starting in the late twentieth century. In other words, the rock-solid faith that PMS is an actual condition is pretty much a Western idea, and it's only in America that PMDD has been officially recognized as an illness. Whereas the Food and Drug Administration accepts PMDD as a disease, the World Health Organization does not.

Speaking of anger: while any premenstrual outburst may be upsetting to us and to those around us, for other women, those few days may actually give them a welcome opportunity to express frustrations that they may not otherwise feel free in venting. Sarafem's slogan is "More like the woman you are." But, excuse us . . . who's to say that "the women we are" don't get incredibly pissed off once in a while, especially if we've been holding it in all month? As Roseanne Barr once said, "Women complain about PMS, but I think of it as the only time of the month when I can be myself."

One thing rarely mentioned by anyone is the fact that for many women, the premenstrual week isn't just a time of nasty mood swings and unexplained tears; it can be a time of great energy, creativity, and focus. It can also be a time of reflection and inwardness. Biologists in Kenya discovered that in their premenstrual days, female baboons regularly seek solitude. Funnily enough, the male baboons don't seem to care or even notice.

And who knows, maybe being cyclically moody is part of our human nature. In 1996, two researchers named Heather Nash and Joan Crisler came up with a study in which they listed classic symptoms of PMS, but replaced the term with the gender-neutral Episodic Dysphoric Disorder. A surprising number of men felt that they suffered from it, and their female friends agreed with them.

In her book *Periods*, Sharon Golub makes the point that we as a culture don't think that being variable is normal; we cling instead to the belief that being the same all the time is normal.

But is it?

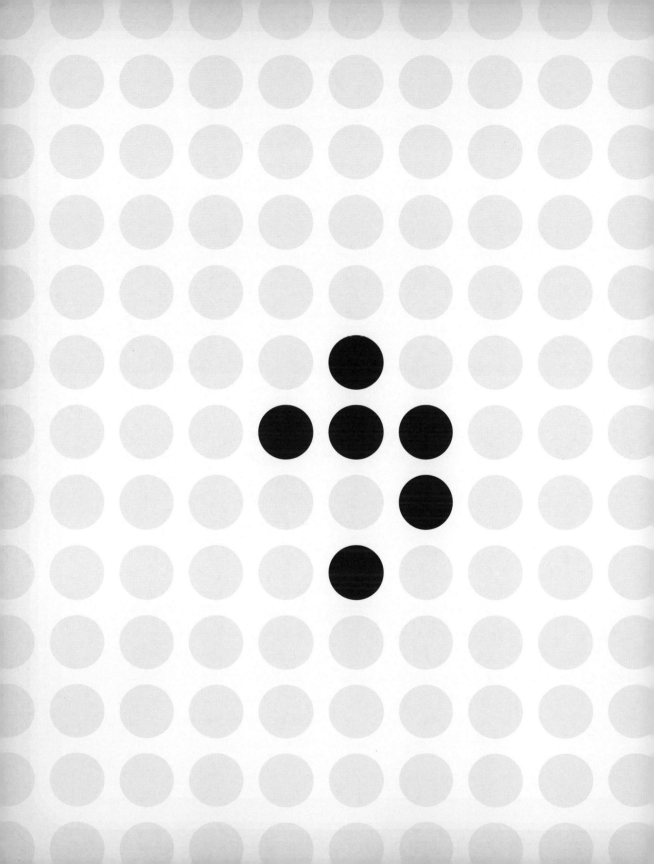

Chapter 6

SEX AND RELIGION

IN 1953, A SMALL, HARD-COVERED BOMB WITH a dust jacket went off in bookstores across America. It was the publication of *Sexual Behavior in the Human Female*, the wildly controversial sex study written by Dr. Alfred Kinsey, Wardell Pomeroy, and their colleagues. Sure, Kinsey & Co. had published *Sexual Behavior in the Human Male* five years earlier, but heck, *that* was no big news; men were *supposed* to like sex! Yet in the very same year that Patti Paige was scoring jukebox gold with "How Much Is That Doggie in the Window?" and Disney's *Peter Pan* was raking in big bucks at the box office, Kinsey's study of actual female sexual practices rocked the horrified country with its candid revelations about sexual fantasies, sadomasochism, lesbianism and bisexuality, childhood sexual urges and experiences, masturbation, and pre- and extra-marital affairs.

Yet for all the unprecedented candor and open-mindedness as its authors traipsed dutifully from one forbidden topic to another, *Sexual Behavior in the Human Female* had virtually nothing to say about menstruation. The interviewers didn't ask their subjects about sex during their periods, nor did any of the women questioned offer any of their own opinions or experiences: how they felt about it, how they dealt with it, or whether or not it was a problem, an excuse, something that was repellent or even a turn-on in the bedroom.

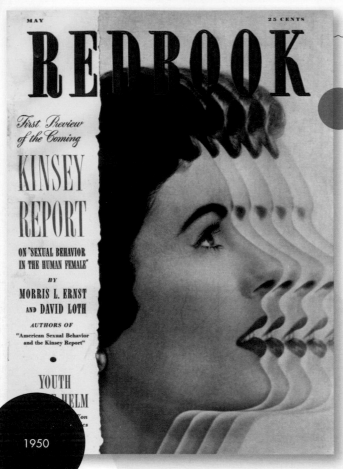

Similarly, *The Hite Report on Female Sexuality* (1976), the first research project about women's sexuality that was conducted by women, was also eerily silent on the subject. In interviewing a hundred thousand women and girls, author Shere Hite uncovered fundamental societal misconceptions about the nature of female sexuality involving frigidity, masturbation, and that whole clitoral-versus-vaginal-stimulation-during-intercourse debate. Yet as progressive and revelatory as it still is today, *The Hite Report* didn't mention sex during menstruation either. Not even once.

And this strikes us as kind of weird.

After all, every female of childbearing age *does* menstruate approximately four to five days every four weeks. What's more, people *do* have sex, so would it be so crazy to predict that the two events might occasionally overlap? So what are we to make of these two highly regarded sex studies avoiding the subject altogether, either consciously or unconsciously? Does that leave us to assume that *all* Americans share the notion that sex is a total nonstarter during a woman's period? Or perhaps that it's one of the deepest sexual taboos of all . . . so deep, it wouldn't occur to either interviewer or subject to even give it a passing mention?

We know that most ancient cultures around the world and throughout history have held negative views about menstruation, to put it mildly. The mysterious, cyclical bleeding of women that arose from neither injury or illness was considered totally freakish even in relatively enlightened times and was more often than not routinely used to demonize women and remind them of their lowly, inferior (yet oddly dangerous) status.

Not surprisingly, men in ancient times had an especially hard time wrapping their minds around the very idea of sex with a menstruating woman. The aversion and fears were so incredibly deeply rooted, the act is referred to in ancient religious and mythology texts—and yet invariably as the source of dire, cosmic mischief.

In Vedic mythology, the great god Vishnu had the bad sense to lie with the goddess Earth when she was menstruating; as a result, she gave birth to monsters that nearly destroyed the planet. Ancient Romans believed that Vulcan, the god of fire and metal-smithing, suffered from birth defects because his mother was menstruating during his conception. And in one of the ancient apocrypha (religious texts written around the same time as but not formally accepted into the Old Testament), it mentions in 2 Esdras, chapter 5: "And menstruous women shall bring forth monsters."

And why do we call menstruation the "curse," anyway? Ask most people and they'll point you to the Bible. It's right there in Genesis, they'll say confidently, as clear as day: Eve's punishment for succumbing to the temptation of the serpent is to be cursed with menstruation. Funnily enough, that's not actually the case. Nowhere in the Bible is it mentioned that her curse involves anything remotely resembling monthly blood. And yet since that's how most people choose to remember the story of Adam and Eve, that's how menstruation received its charming—and theologically loaded—nickname.

While Christians blame the first woman for the subsequent moral downfall of humankind—and all for one lousy apple, for crying out loud!—the inherent baseness of women echoes thematically throughout other early religions, as well. Ecclesiasticus 25:19 has this to say about the fair sex: "No wickedness comes anywhere

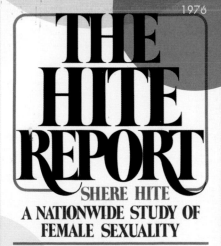

1976

THE HITE REPORT

SHERE HITE

A NATIONWIDE STUDY OF FEMALE SEXUALITY

3,000 women, ages 14 to 78, describe in their own words their most intimate feelings about sex including:
- What they like—and don't like
- How orgasm really feels—with and without intercourse
- How it feels not to have an orgasm during sex
- The importance of clitoral stimulation and masturbation
- And, the greatest pleasures and frustrations of their sexual lives

With a new cultural interpretation of female sexuality

Macmillan Publishing Company

near the wickedness of a woman." From 25:24: "Sin began with a woman and thanks to her, we all must die." And from 22:3: "The birth of a daughter is a loss." Nice, huh? And even today, Orthodox Jewish men still recite a daily prayer, "Blessed art Thou, Lord our God, King of the Universe, who hast not made me a woman."

In much of the Islamic world and among Hindus in India, women must still adhere to the strict rules of purdah, which literally means "curtain." According to purdah, men aren't allowed to see women—who, while in public, must always be covered in a loose, floor-length burka, and with a yashmak, or veil, frequently covering their face, as well. In accordance with this practice, a woman's social and economic activities outside her home are seriously curtailed, and even within her own home, she is often physically segregated from the men with high-walled enclosures, screens, and curtains.

Clearly, women (representing temptation, weakness, and immorality) have long meant trouble with a capital *T* in many world religions, but when they're actually *menstruating*—Katie, bar the door! Consider Leviticus 15:19–23, which sets forth the ancient doctrine of menstrual cooties in no uncertain terms:

> *If a woman has a discharge, and the discharge from her body is blood, she shall be set apart seven days; and whoever touches her shall be unclean until evening. Everything that she lies on during her impurity shall be unclean; also everything that she sits on shall be unclean. Whoever touches her bed shall wash his clothes and bathe in water, and be unclean until evening. And whoever touches anything that she sat on shall wash his clothes and bathe in water, and be unclean until evening. If anything is on her bed or on anything on which she sits, when he touches it, he shall be unclean until evening.*

And that, my friends, is some serious uncleanliness! This sentiment is echoed in the Koran, 2:222: "They ask thee concerning women's courses. Say: They are a hurt and a pollution: So keep away from women in their courses, and do not approach them until they are clean." Similarly, in Eastern Hinduism, a menstruating woman is forbidden from taking part in religious ceremonies for the first four days of her cycle. And in ancient India, sex was also forbidden during her flow.

Yet what was an ancient people to do, what with 50 percent of one's community continually spending so much time wallowing in their own filth, corrupting everything they touched and being a loathsome abomination in general? One couldn't exactly banish women *all* the time—who else could the guys turn to for the cooking, harvesting, food storage, cleaning, childcare, and sex?

As a result, many religions and cultures cleverly devised ritualized cleansing ceremonies to regularly purge women of their monthly impurities—rites that still continue in many parts of the world to this day. Not only do such rituals assuage the male fear

In the Bible, a woman used to be allowed to cleanse herself every month symbolically, with animal sacrifices.

of contamination, allowing a man to enjoy his wife's charms and services with a clear conscience, but by establishing a cycle of filth and cleansing made up of ritualized banishment and reacceptance, male-dominated society perpetuates the cozy myth that women are flawed, dirty, and routinely in need of being made clean again. The implication becomes that women not only *deserve* the treatment they receive, in fact, they're pretty damn lucky!

In certain Islamic sects, women must perform a ritual cleansing bath, a *ghusl*, washing themselves thoroughly from head to toe, making sure their hair and scalp are scrubbed clean, as well. The *Manusmriti* (one of the foundations of Hindu law) also requires ritual bathing at every cycle's conclusion.

In the Bible, a woman used to be allowed to cleanse herself every month symbolically, with animal sacrifices; just check out Leviticus 15:29–30: "And on the eighth day she shall take unto her two turtledoves, or two young pigeons, and bring them unto the priest, to the door of the tabernacle of the congregation. And the priest shall offer the one for a sin offering, and the other for a burnt offering; and the priest shall make an atonement for her before the Lord for the issue of her uncleanness." But given animal rights and anticruelty laws (not to mention the going price of turtledoves and pigeons), that's no longer a viable option. Instead, there's always the mikvah—perhaps the best-known and most controversial ritual, intended for many purifying uses for both men and women, but best known for postmenstrual cleansing.

To understand the mikvah, one needs to understand the female cycle, according to Orthodox Jews. The Talmud (the interpretation of the Hebrew Bible by ancient rabbis and scholars) added another week following the end of the period, which means that a Jewish woman—at least according to Orthodox rules—is considered unclean for at least two weeks out of the month. During this time, she is *niddah*. This means "separated," referring specifically to any physical contact with her husband. And "separated" means no hugging, no hand-holding, no casual brushing a stray crumb off his chin, and most certainly no sex, for half of the month.

In order to begin the purification process, a woman must wait until seven days after the last day of her period. Then she checks herself internally for any trace of blood. Using a small, clean, white cloth (special ones called *bedikah* are made for this purpose), she checks the vaginal canal to make sure it's blood-free. Alternatively, she could opt to wear white underwear and sleep on white sheets. When everything is completely free from even the faintest trace of menstrual flow, she's finally ready to be spiritually cleansed.

First, the woman bathes, shampoos and combs her hair, and removes anything touching or covering her skin: watches, jewelry, makeup, even bandages. She often undoes any braids, as well, to ensure that every bit of her, including each filament of hair, will be totally immersed. The mikvah itself has been built into the ground, in its own house or as an integral part of another building. It is filled according to strict rabbinical law; and when a woman steps into it, the waters must completely envelop her body. After reciting a purification blessing, she dunks herself two more times. And only after she has completed this ritual can she get back to connubial relations with her husband.

In clinical terms, one can well see the advantages of such a setup when it comes to population growth: after two weeks of abstinence without so much as a furtive hand squeeze, a woman is suddenly free to be with her husband at the height of ovulation, thus standing a pretty good chance of getting pregnant.

However, this practicality is just an extra bonus tacked on to an ancient and disturbing belief: that menstrual sex is contaminating and must be systematically cleansed. From early Christian clergy such as Pope Dionysius of Alexandria (d. A.D. 265): "Menstruous women ought not to come to the Holy Table, or touch the Holy of Holies, nor to churches, but pray elsewhere." From Saint Theodore, seventh Archbishop of Canterbury (d. A.D. 690), who centralized the English Church: "During the time of menstruation women should not enter into church or receive communion, neither lay women nor religious." The whammy was apparently on women even when they weren't actually bleeding, as witnessed by this remark by Theodulf, Bishop of Orléans (d. A.D. 821): "While a priest is celebrating Mass, women should in no way approach the altar, but remain in their places, and there the priest should receive their offerings to God. Women should therefore remember their infirmity, and the inferiority of their sex: and therefore they should have fear of touching whatever sacred things there are in the ministry of the Church."

Today, religion and menstruation are still, so to speak, uncomfortable bed partners—witness Pope Benedict's visit to Poland in 2006. Deemed by lily-livered broadcasters as "inappropriate," all ads for tampons—along with those for beer and lingerie—were banned from the air on state TV during his stay.

Oddly enough, religious squeamishness about menstruation wasn't always monolithic; there were even some rare moments of enlightenment. In certain branches of Buddhism, for instance, menstruation has always been seen as something natural. Any overt sexism, such as the banning of women from temples, has been interpreted by some as a later influence of Hinduism.

Even representing the Church, Pope Gregory I wrote, in A.D. 601: "The natural flux that she suffers cannot be imputed to her as a fault, therefore it is right that she should not be deprived of the entrance into a church." He also wrote that while a menstruating woman who preferred to remain outside a church should be praised, her condition still shouldn't be held against her; and should she choose to enter, she shouldn't be punished.

We find it distressing that this bit of humane common sense was considered so revolutionary, especially considering that Jesus himself was famously empathetic to at least one woman who was menstruating. From Matthew 9:20–22: "Just then a woman who had been subject to bleeding for twelve years came up behind him and touched the edge of his cloak. She said to herself, 'If I only touch his cloak, I will be healed.' Jesus turned and saw her. 'Take heart, daughter,' he said, 'your faith has healed you.' And the woman was healed from that moment." While we may initially be stunned by the idea of any woman bleeding for twelve years, we are more impressed by Jesus' radical behavior. Not only does he clearly not care a snap of his fingers about possible contamination by contact with the poor woman, he also heals what sounds like a runaway case of menorrhagia, or excessive menstrual flow.

Religious taboos against menstruation still persist. Orthodox Jewish men won't

Orthodox Jewish men won't shake hands with a woman for fear she may be menstruating, thus rendering him impure.

shake hands with a woman for fear she may be menstruating, thus rendering him impure. In the Talmud it is stated that if a menstruating woman walks between two men, one of them will die (leaving us to ponder what world history would have been like if we had actually had that kind of power all along . . . the mind reels!). In Jerusalem, a special bus system for the very religious ensures that by seating the men up front and women in back, no chance contamination might occur. In his 2007 book, *The Year of*

Living Biblically, author A. J. Jacobs realized it was virtually impossible in New York City to sit anywhere that a menstruating woman definitely hadn't been, and so had to resort to carrying a folding chair with him everywhere he went.

According to Islam, menstruating women are still forbidden to touch the Koran, perform special prayers at Islamic festivals, fast (being expected to make up the days at other times during the year), and, last but not least, have sex with their husbands. According to the Koran: "When they have purified themselves, ye may approach them in any manner, time, or place ordained for you by God. For God loves those who turn to Him constantly and He loves those who keep themselves pure and clean."

"All right," we hear you say, "we get it. World religions have always been run by men, and any religious beliefs and rituals about menstruation are little more than ancient superstitions based on primitive fears, none of which have any place in the twenty-first century. After all, except for a distinct minority of the religiously conservative and very devout, no one actually believes any of this menstrual sex/pollution nuttiness anymore . . . do they?"

The creepy thing is, they do and they don't.

If one is up for a mirthless laugh or two, we suggest visiting any of the consumer-oriented Web sites maintained by the big femcare manufacturers. One and all, the sites address myths we're depressed to hear apparently still need debunking, notions that many females obviously still cling to, such as: Is it safe to wash one's hair during one's period? Is it okay to take a bath? And from the Barr Pharmaceuticals–sponsored Web site, knowyourperiods.com: Is menstrual blood poisonous? Is sex with a menstruating woman dangerous? Admittedly, Pliny the Edler wrote that sex with a menstruating woman during a solar or lunar eclipse could be fatal. But remember, he came up with that one in A.D. 60. How weird is it that many of us are clearly still haunted by menstrual superstitions dating back for literally thousands of years?

The Internet, being the clearinghouse of not only much useful information but also rants from the fringe, gives us this recent mature post from a mainstream men's health Web site: "Some guys are absolutely disgusted at the mere thought of going anywhere near her vagina when it should be 'closed for maintenance,' " and guys should explore other ways to be satisfied "until her playground's no longer muddy." Such sentiments eerily echo those of 1951's *The Illustrated Encyclopedia of Sex*, which stated that both men and women were often queasy about female genitalia even when a woman wasn't menstruating, "because of the wetness of the zone. They think it is messy, or that a woman is 'dirtier' than a man."

All right, already; we think we've succeeded in making ourselves seriously depressed. It's time for a much-needed reality check, okay?

Despite all the apparent squeamishness out there, many women and their partners in fact find sex during menstruation just ducky. Sure, one can still get pregnant in the process if not using protection, and what's more, it might not be the best time to break out those 500-thread-count Egyptian pima sheets. Some women keep an extra set of dark sheets or a towel on hand to deal with the spillage. Others shrug and say to hell with it.

Some women also find their mojo runs a bit higher during their periods. Even the

> **Did you know that both sex and orgasms help relieve menstrual cramps? What's more, the uterine contractions of orgasm help propel one's flow on its journey down and out, always a good thing. And oxytocin, often called the "bonding" or "love" hormone, is routinely released during orgasm, bringing with it a much-welcome sense of calm and well-being. What could be better when one is perhaps feeling a tad bloated and achey in the first place?**

otherwise dour *Illustrated Encyclopedia of Sex* grudgingly admits that menstruation might have some sort of influence on a woman's sex drive ("a nervous excitability that considerably affects their mood and conduct"), albeit not necessarily a positive one. And last but not least, a 2002 study done at Yale University indicates that women who have orgasms during menstruation are less likely to develop endometriosis. How's that for encouraging?

So where does all this leave menstruation, sex, and religion today? We're intrigued to report that there are people out there willing to push the envelope a little, such as those who follow Tantrism. This faith, which started in ancient India, features sex rites and ceremonies that throw traditional, male-centric, and subordinate roles for women out the window. Both male and female bodies are celebrated equally, as are fertility and sex. In fact, the highest of Tantric sexual rites calls for a menstruating woman to be an active participant.

Thousands of Jewish women are also reclaiming the mikvah—transforming it into a positive personal and spiritual experience. Whether to acknowledge a significant life change, a happy event, or a personal loss, women are connecting to the regeneration and rebirth symbolism of immersion in a completely new way, although not necessarily to the liking of the more traditionally minded in the Jewish community.

Okay, we're not saying the world will be saved by people reinventing the mikvah or practicing Tantric sex (although the idea does intrigue). Yet sex and religion, at least as they relate to menstruation, have been extraordinarily powerful for centuries, reinforcing negative and damaging mistruths about women and their bodies that linger to this day. Making a stand for the basic rights of women may start with something as simple as questioning where such taboos come from . . . and beginning to eradicate those powerful religious stigmas that make menstruation such a dirty word in the first place.

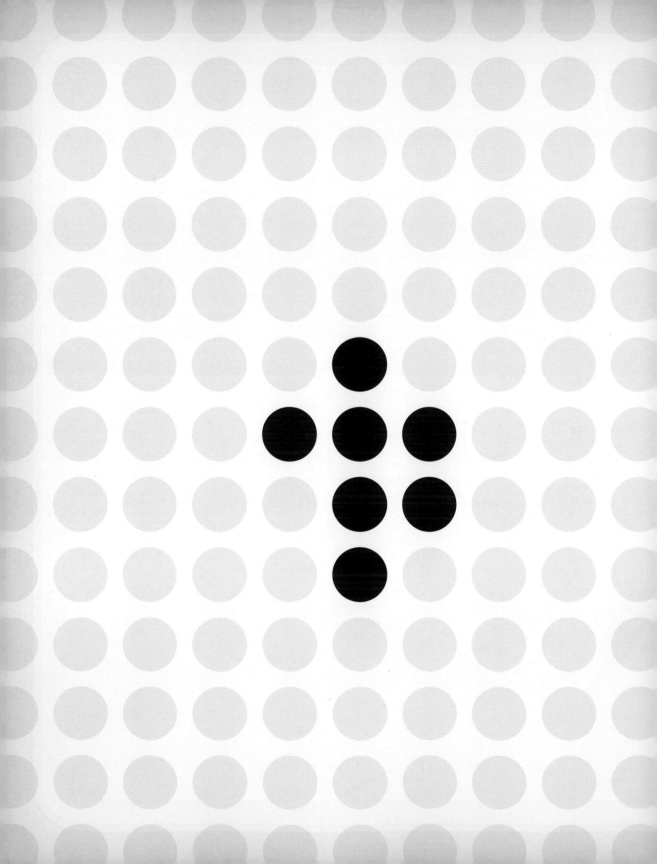

Chapter 7

SOCIETY'S ROLE

ACCORDING TO STUDIES, ONE OUT OF EVERY TEN school-age girls in today's sub-Sarahan Africa routinely skips school when she has her period or just drops out altogether once she hits puberty. This is due to lack of not only private facilities (and it can be traumatic enough to go change a tampon in eighth grade even with the most private bathroom in the world), but basic femcare, as well. Added up, these absences total something like 10 to 20 percent of missed school time, which puts the average African schoolgirl at a huge disadvantage for the rest of her life. As a result, in November 2007, Procter & Gamble brands Always and Tampax announced that they were teaming up with HERO, an initiative of the United Nations Association. Their five-year awareness-building program is called Protecting Futures, through which, along with improving education, nutrition, and health services, they plan to distribute free Always and Tampax products to a small network of schools. "There are lots of reasons kids miss school," said the P&G director of the program. "Being a girl shouldn't be one of them."

Commercial femcare is not unlike clothing in that both share a strange relationship with the social and political movements of the day. Developments and innovations in both have not only reflected society but, like all good design, have arisen directly and organically from the needs, beliefs, and values of the times. As a result, even the lowly pad or the humblest tampon can claim to be a genuine, if unconventional, agent of change.

Here in today's America, we tend to be downright blasé about the social, political, and career opportunities available to us as women. While there may still be a glass ceiling, we only notice it because we're finally high enough to bump against it. Nobody bats an eye at the thought of a female tennis champion, prime minister, astrophysicist, hedge fund manager, baseball ump, or lead guitarist. Women are not only capable of bringing home the bacon and frying it up in a pan, we can also marry and divorce at will, stay single and/or childless without being burned as some kind of witch, take out mortgages, own property, control our own money, pursue a Ph.D., and vote. Along the way, we can buy tampons, too. Yet a mere hundred years ago, virtually none of this was even a remote possibility.

Since its inception, the struggle for women's rights has been and continues to be like a pendulum swinging back and forth between progress and reaction to that progress. Funnily enough, the two most important women's movements of American history also happened to coincide with the biggest gains in menstrual management. Hard-fought gains in women's rights came about just as advances in femcare were promising and actually creating new and unheard-of opportunities.

Conveniently, the movement for women's rights can be broken down into three waves. "First-wave feminism" took place during the late nineteenth and early twentieth centuries in the United States and United Kingdom. It concerned itself in part with some pretty radical and wild-eyed notions: that women could, for example, own property all by themselves, have sex without being married, exercise birth control, and not be literally owned, along with their children, by their husbands and fathers like so much furniture. Mostly, however, first-wave feminism was about female suffrage—the right to vote.

Back then, there was a lot more at stake to voting rights than just being allowed to wear goofy campaign buttons, pull a lever, and then watch election returns on CNN with a sinking stomach. The underlying argument—that women were actually entitled to basic rights as individuals outside of their standing with men—became a prickly, nay, downright cranky national debate. In fact (and you may want to sit down for this part), most believed that a woman's menstrual cycle made her inherently unstable, irresponsible, and incapable of any kind of intellectual rigor, a virtual time bomb of tears, soggy emotionalism, and hysteria.

The New York Times, the esteemed Gray Lady herself, published this opinion in 1912: "No doctor can ever lose sight of the fact that the mind of a woman is always threatened with danger from the reverberations of her physiological emergencies (i.e., menstruation). It is with such thoughts that the doctor lets his eyes rest upon the militant suffragist. He cannot shut them to the fact that there is mixed up in the woman's movement such mental disorder, and he cannot conceal from himself the physiological emergencies which lie behind." And the year before: "The mind of woman is so essentially different from that of man. Are you prepared to introduce sentimentalism and hysteria into the most solemn task a freeman has to execute—a task which should be approached

Funnily enough, the two most important women's movements of American history also happened to coincide with the biggest gains in menstrual management.

1913

in the same spirit in which you would approach a church—a task calling for the best powers of a mature masculine mind?"

Early suffrage workers like Lucy Burns and Alice Paul, founders of the National Woman's Party (NWP), didn't have the luxury of fronting a movement from a comfy home office, armed with the Internet, an espresso machine, and some landlines. They instead held rallies, wrote pamphlets, organized parades, protested in front of the White House, chained themselves to fences, and went on hunger strikes . . . and as a direct result, were summarily beaten, shackled, arrested, thrown in prison, and, once there, tortured apparently for the sheer heck of it. And has one ever wondered throughout all this how these women actually handled getting their periods on top of everything else? Come to think of it, what did any woman do, prior to the advent of commercial femcare, in order to manage her monthly blood?

The answer, such as it is, will make you blanch. Up until a hundred years ago, women had to sling together their own methods of dealing with their flow any ol' way they could—with rags, towels, or with nothing at all. All of this seriously limited their mobility, meaning it was a pretty dire time for women's freedom, both literally and figuratively. As for the suffrage workers, almost nothing has been recorded about how they dealt with their menstrual flow—as it was, a woman's right to vote only barely merited serious mention in the press, so one can only imagine how such august publications as the *Times* felt about something as essentially ignominious as blood regularly seeping from female loins.

One thing that made the problem of femcare back then so incredibly challenging, a puzzler worthy of Einstein, was the lack of underwear. Ever wonder about the illustrious history of that microfiber thong of yours? Back in the nineteenth century, there were no panties, undies, bikinis, briefs, boy shorts, nary even a set of knickers. For centuries, undergarments weren't about hygiene or propriety, but rather artificiality, adornment, and warmth: chemises, petticoats, rib-cracking corsets, bodices.

Perhaps one reason for all those petticoats and shifts was to protect one's outer dress from blood and other stains . . . or perhaps we kid ourselves. After all, if one was industrious and had a little mad money, it was possible to scare up a cotton apron lined with rubber, which presumably kept blood from seeping into the seat of one's dress. There were also bloomers with rubber panels at the bottom available; but all of these were relative rarities, and due to their cost, effectively out of range for most women. No, most had to resort to stuffing between their legs or up their vaginas those materials they could get for free: rags, pieces of sheepskin, leaves, moss, or nothing at all.

From Harry Finley, founder of the online Museum of Menstruation, comes this translation from Friedrich Eduard Bilz's *Das Neue Naturheilverfahren* (*The New Natural Healing*), published in the late nineteenth century: "Many women . . . place

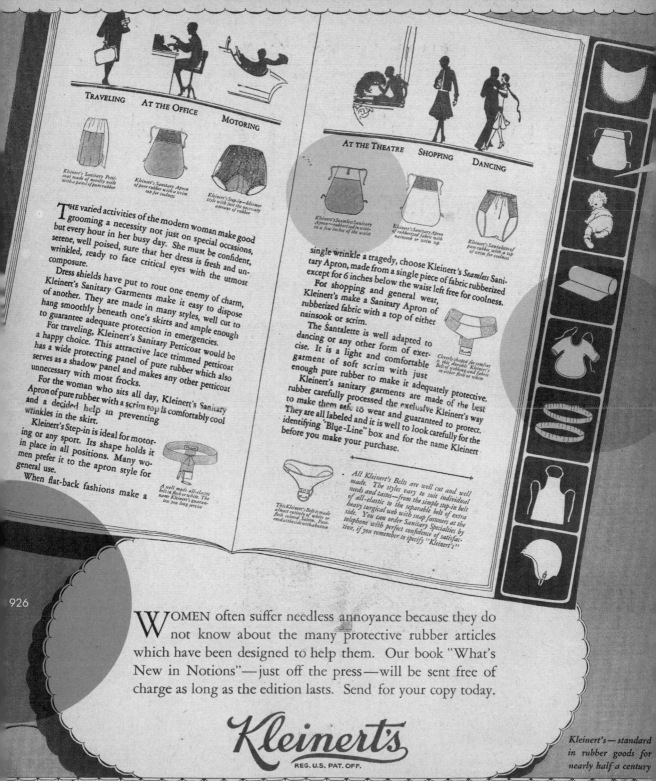

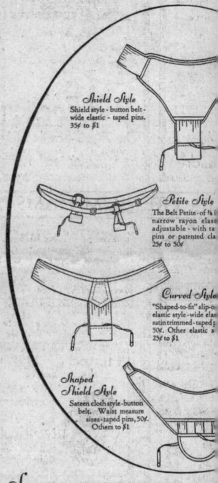

nothing in that region [to absorb menses] and so in addition to the outer sex organs, underwear, sheets and bed covers, the lower belly and thighs are stiffened with dried blood . . . and finally because of the widespread prejudice against frequent washing and changing of clothes during this time, some women, even those of the better classes, are often filthy to an almost unbelievable degree." Gives one a whole new way of looking at Scarlett O'Hara and Marie Antoinette, doesn't it?

Women could also depend on the good ol' terra firma, the ground itself. Female factory workers would often work standing up, sans underwear and knee-deep in straw into which they freely bled. The workstation, much like a stall full of farm animals, would be mucked out when the conditions became unbearably filthy.

So it was like a shining knight on a sanitary white charger when manufactured menstrual products hit the marketplace, literally affording a "new freedom" to women. In 1896, Johnson & Johnson introduced the very first disposable pad, Lister's Towels (named for Joseph Lister, a British surgeon who popularized the concept of sterile surgery). To be sure, it took a while for commercial menstrual products to catch on, given what they were and the limits of advertising in such a relatively genteel time. But 1920 finally saw the ratification of the Nineteenth Amendment, which stated: "The right of citizens of the United States to vote shall not be denied or abridged by the United States or by any State on account of sex." And the same year, Kotex pads went on sale.

Commercial femcare products were soon proliferating, and related advertising was up and running, as well. Yet as is the case with any giddy new revolution, there was a certain measure of morning-after reality. Even with all the newfound freedom Kotex promised,

Shield Style
Shield style - button belt - wide elastic - taped pins. 35¢ to $1

Petite Style
The Belt Petite - of ¼ i narrow rayon elast adjustable - with ta pins or patented cla 25¢ to 50¢

Curved Style
"Shaped-to-fit" slip-o elastic style - wide elas satin trimmed - taped p 50¢. Other elastic s 25¢ to $1

Shaped Shield Style
Sateen cloth style - button belt. Waist measure sizes - taped pins, 50¢. Others to $1

SKETCHED ABOVE are but four of the many different popu varieties of BELTS by HICKORY—always dependable, yet gently cure. Ask your dealer for style and size you prefer. You can depend up it, it will be a new delight and revelation in comfort. Never binds or co strains. HICKORY BELTS are approved and recommended by leadi medical authorities. Ask your physician . . . Buy a HICKORY and y own a world of comfort. . . . .TO BE HAD at your favorite sto early disposable pads were no walk in the park. They were bulky, uncomfortable, cumbersome, and had to be attached, with safety pins or clips, to elastic belts that one wore around the waist. The whole getup was unwieldy and annoying, with major slippage potential, not to mention many opportunities for sudden, unexpected leaking. In the 1930s, commercial tampons were introduced, and they, too, were beset by problems, being clunky, awkward to insert, and not even especially absorbent. Still, these early prototypes at least beat bleeding into one's crummy petticoat, and early-twentieth-century women must have surely basked in the heady glow of this fledgling political and menstrual freedom.

But at the same time, society was sneakily working on its own covert agenda. Guess what was introduced the year after women won the right to vote and Kotex hit the stores? The Miss America beauty pageant. Coincidence? From the very start, as if in direct if unconscious response to all those sweaty, noisy, totally undainty suffrage workers, the pageant championed an old-fashioned ideal of femininity. Racy, bobbed haircuts were forbidden, as was any makeup. In fact, anything modern was verboten in the fledgling pageant world, until at last the prototype of Miss America emerged as the squeaky clean, idealized representation of womanhood she is today . . . still conveying the message that despite any achievements or education, the ideal woman is still, above all, demure and decorative. And while Miss America's unflagging popularity held steady for years (its annual televised extravaganza was consistently top-rated from its first airing in 1951 through much of the 1960s), conflict was bubbling elsewhere under society's seemingly placid surface.

In 1963, *The Feminine Mystique* landed in bookstores, and overnight, Betty Friedan tore a new hole in the illusion that women were fulfilled being merely wives, moth-

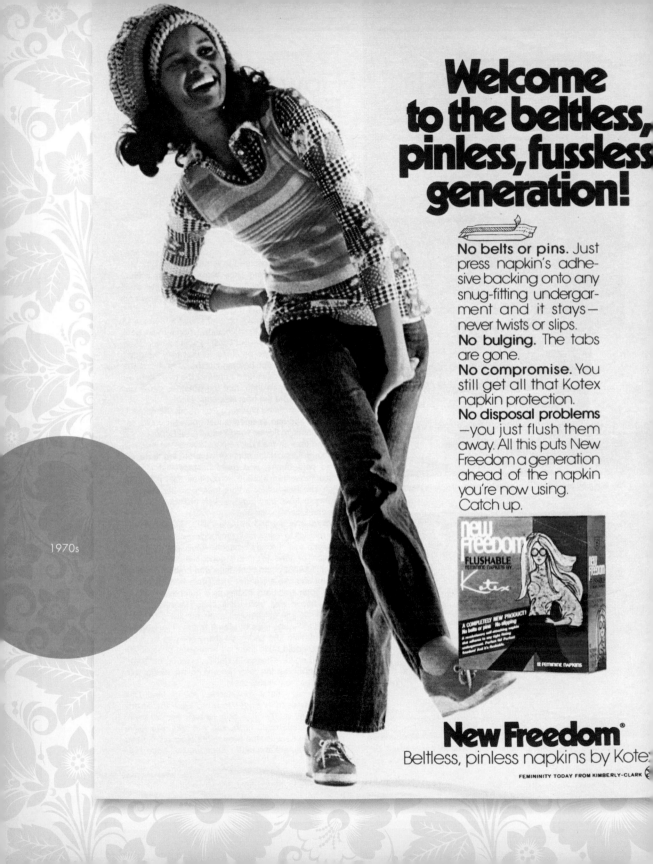

Welcome to the beltless, pinless, fussless generation!

No belts or pins. Just press napkin's adhesive backing onto any snug-fitting undergarment and it stays—never twists or slips.
No bulging. The tabs are gone.
No compromise. You still get all that Kotex napkin protection.
No disposal problems —you just flush them away. All this puts New Freedom a generation ahead of the napkin you're now using. Catch up.

New Freedom®
Beltless, pinless napkins by Kotex

FEMININITY TODAY FROM KIMBERLY-CLARK

1970s

ers, and homemakers. In the first chapter, "The Problem That Has No Name," she wrote: "The problem lay buried, unspoken, for many years in the minds of American women. . . . As she made the beds, shopped for groceries, matched slipcover material, ate peanut butter sandwiches with her children, chauffeured Cub Scouts and Brownies, lay beside her husband at night—she was afraid to ask even of herself the silent question—'Is this all?'"

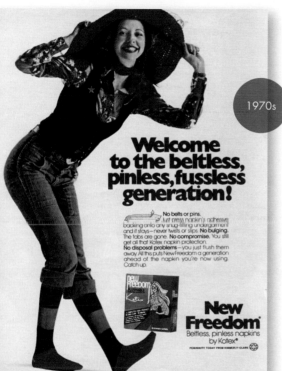

While there were certainly many women who felt Friedan got it all wrong, still others who felt trapped by domesticity found in her message both a kindred spirit and a rallying cry. Thus, the so-called second wave of feminism was launched. With the vote long since sewn up, the women's liberation movement protested fundamental inequalities and championed everything from parity in wages and the Equal Rights Amendment to fair access to education and abortion rights. Birth control pills became available in the early 1960s, women's health collectives sprang up as an alternative to the male-dominated medical establishment, and the first edition of that estimable alternative women's health bible, *Our Bodies, Ourselves*, came out in 1973. Midwives came back into fashion and the number of natural childbirths rocketed.

Title IX was passed in 1972, which meant schools could no longer discriminate when it came to funding and providing sports and activities for girls. Women's rights took another significant leap forward in 1973 when the Supreme Court heard *Roe v. Wade* and legalized abortion in all fifty states, ruling that privacy regarding one's reproductive system was consistent with the Fourteenth Amendment to the United States Constitution. And while all this was going on, self-adhesive sanitary napkins hit the market.

Not a big deal, you say? Oh, ho-ho . . . but we beg to differ.

Overnight, restrictive menstrual gear, practically the same kind one's grandmother had to use—goofy sanitary belts, safety pins and clips, special panties, oversize pads—became singularly obsolete, a thing of the past. With names like New Freedom, Carefree, and Stayfree, it was clear that change was in the air, baby!

Since pads no longer needed to be superlong to be anchored to those clips fore and aft, they were given permission to shrink. What's more, superabsorbent materials were developed, allowing pad makers to make their product even slimmer and lighter—and far less detectable—than before. New products, like minipads, were invented and became all the rage.

But as women fought discrimination in the workplace and society, there simultaneously developed an unmistakable feminist trend toward negating the feminine, as well. This is when the women's movement took on all those unsavory "man-hating" connotations that unfortunately linger to this day.

To be fair, there probably was a lot going on along those lines back then. Come to think of it, who could blame women for militantly refusing to come in second anymore, no matter what the price? Yet anything that smacked even faintly of the feminine or girly was soon seen as suspect, even downright counterrevolutionary. Lipstick, anything pink, and being a housewife were viewed with an equally hairy eyeball, whereas navy business suits, big shoulder pads, and not shaving or wearing makeup were suddenly de rigeur. Overnight, Everywoman became Superwoman, implying there was something deeply wrong with you if you couldn't have it all and do it all. The party line evolved that women were not just equal to but the same as or even better than men: a position that came close to negating biology and natural differences.

Similarly, anything that had to do with menstruation was often disparaged, in some cases even eliminated. In 1971, a feminist reproductive health self-help group came up with a do-it-yourself "period extraction kit," by which one's entire period could be hoovered out in mere minutes. Women were urged to get together with a few friends, hop up on the dining room table, and practice extracting each other's periods. The inventors toured the country, demonstrating the technique at women-only seminars.

As eyebrow-raising as it may seem now, it was surprisingly, if briefly, *le dernier cri* as a fad, not unlike goldfish swallowing or piling into a telephone booth.

And where are we today?

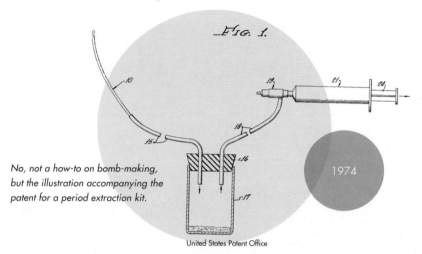

No, not a how-to on bomb-making, but the illustration accompanying the patent for a period extraction kit.

United States Patent Office

PATENTED MENSTRUAL PRODUCTS THAT DIDN'T SET THE WORLD ON FIRE

- A tampon that would let the wearer know when it was almost filled to capacity (patent #7,214,848—2001)

- An intravaginal balloon that would prevent any leaking (patent #6,747,184—2004)

- A tampon with an adhesive string that would prevent it from being seen when wearing a bathing suit (patent #6,679,868—2001)

- A vulvar deodorant system (patent #3,948,257—1976)

- A sanitary napkin with a rear strip that would reside in the user's intergluteal crevice, aka one's butt crack (patent #6,613,031—2003)

Well, from the early 1990s onward, we've been told that we're hip-deep in feminism's third wave. So what exactly are today's feminists fighting for? After all, women already have the right to vote, and in many areas, discrimination and inequality have been, if not eliminated, then at least reduced. Reproductive rights have become a different battlefield with the advent of RU-486, and to make things even more complicated, there's no longer anything approaching consensus on the ethical nuances of abortion and choice.

What's more, there's been a generational reaction against feminism's second wave, which was in fact created by and geared toward middle-class, white, college-educated women. The second wave didn't pretend to represent minorities, or touch on vital global, class, or sexuality issues. The third-wave feminist issues seem to be more about individual empowerment and personal decisions about everything from consumer choices to sexual expression than they are about any single, overriding ideology of what it means to be female. Perhaps appropriately, commercial femcare also appears to be riding something of a third wave, as well.

Thanks to menstrual suppression drugs, we can now choose how often we menstruate, if at all. Yet this raises numerous questions, from health risks to problems with potential fertility. And we wonder: Is this one giant leap forward for womankind, freedom from hormonal shifts, bleeding, the risk of unplanned pregnancy? Or a step backward—that by ridding ourselves of an intrinsic part of being female, we're trying to make ourselves more like men? Are all periods a problem and is ending them genuine empowerment? Or is this just another shrewd, shortsighted corporate ploy based on making us hate our own bodies?

We're raising a generation of girls for whom girl power is taken for granted, and so maybe it's no surprise that this is where we are. In essence, we're handing young women the opportunity to change the way their bodies work, erasing something that's been a fundamental female experience since the first humans stood up from all that primordial goo. While we believe women should be free to do what they want with their bodies, we're nevertheless disturbed by the underlying message being sold to us wholesale, no questions asked . . . and all for a lousy buck.

Sure, it's progress. We're just wondering if it's in the right direction.

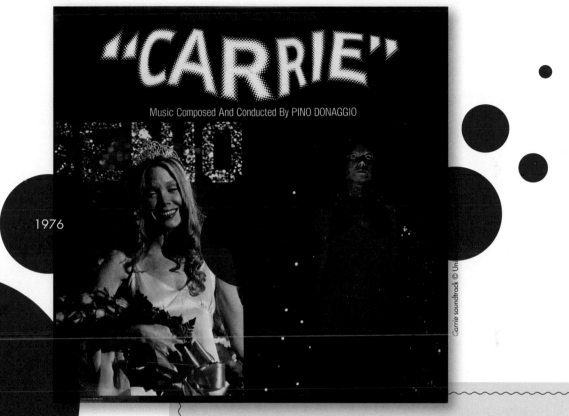

"CARRIE"

Music Composed And Conducted By PINO DONAGGIO

1976

Carrie soundtrack © Uni

MENSTRUATION IN THE MOVIES

Carrie, directed in 1976 by Brian De Palma and based on the Stephen King novel, is a suburban horror movie about menstruation, the taboos surrounding it, and the power it can unleash. High school loser Carrie White is the butt of the school's derision when she gets her first period in gym class; but woe to all those who mock her at the prom! To some, it's a cheesy camp-fest; to us, it's one of the best horror films ever made, a true fairy tale for grown-ups and an extraordinary meditation on the awesome power of budding female sexuality.

Menstrual

TIME LINE

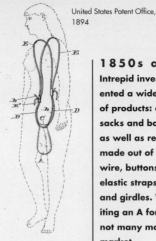

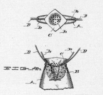

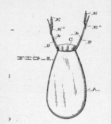

1850s and On

Intrepid inventors patented a wide variety of products: catamenial sacks and bandages, as well as receptacles made out of springs, wire, buttons, flaps, elastic straps, valves, and girdles. While meriting an A for creativity, not many made it to market.

1839

Charles Goodyear invented the technology to vulcanize rubber, which was used in manufacturing rubber condoms, intra-uterine devices, douching syringes, and the "womb veil," aka the diaphragm.

ANCIENT WORLD

Egyptian women used softened papyrus for tampons. In Greece, tampons were rigged out of lint wrapped around small pieces of wood (yeow!), whereas in Rome, pads and tampons were made of soft wool. Women in Japan used paper. Native Americans made tampons out of moss and pads from buffalo skin. Women also used wool, sponges, and grass to absorb their flow.

1934

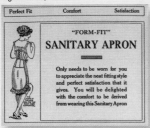

Logan Fabrics, 1920s

Perfect Fit	Comfort	Satisfaction

"FORM-FIT"
SANITARY APRON

Only needs to be worn for you to appreciate the neat fitting style and perfect satisfaction that it gives. You will be delighted with the comfort to be derived from wearing this Sanitary Apron

Early Twentieth Century

Many American women used homemade pads, often rigged out of "bird's eye," the same absorbent cotton material used for baby diapers. They would pin these cloths, or rags, to their underwear or to homemade muslin belts.

Sanitary aprons were available through catalogs. Worn backwards with a rubber shield hanging down over a woman's backside, they protected dress backs from menstrual staining. Not being absorbent, they leave us wondering, where the hell did all the blood go?

Sanitary bloomers were another early product available through the mail. Modeled after diaper covers, they had a rubber panel that kept blood from seeping through one's clothing. They were hot and bulky, not to mention all that trapped moisture brought on untold chafing and infections.

1926

Sanitary bloomers

1896

Lister's Towels, the first commercial sanitary pads, went on sale. Produced by Johnson & Johnson (and named for Joseph Lister, a pioneer in sterile surgery) and arguably too avant-garde for the prudish times, they sank like a proverbial rock.

World War I

When nurses in France realized that the cellulose bandages they were using on wounded soldiers absorbed blood much better than plain old cotton, they started using them for their own flow.

1873

The Comstock Act was passed, making it a federal crime to distribute or sell pornography or conception-related materials or text in the United States. In response, the birth control industry coined the term "feminine hygiene" to advertise their repackaged, over-the-counter products (which generally didn't work, anyway).

1911

Midol, marketed as a remedy for headaches and toothaches, went on sale. Eventually, it would become synonymous with menstrual pain relief.

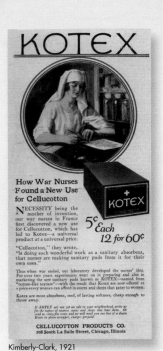

Early 1920s

Kotex (a combination of "cotton" and "texture") landed in stores. Luckily for women everywhere, Kimberly-Clark found an innovative way to use up all those leftover surgical wound dressings after World War I had ended. Who knows what would have happened if there hadn't been a practical need to unload excess inventory?

Mid-1920s

A revolution in fashion: women's underwear became close-crotched! Open crotches had been all the rage, as the design made relieving oneself under all those long layers easier, but a closed crotch was far better for holding a belt and pad in place.

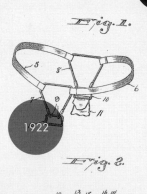

United States Patent Office, 1922

Disposable pads, while a big step forward when it came to convenience, couldn't be worn without reusable sanitary belts. Made of elastic and worn around the waist, a sanitary belt had clips that attached to tabs on the front and back of a pad. Alternatively, women used safety pins to hold the pads in place.

Kimberly-Clark encouraged store owners to display Kotex on their counters, along with a discreet box for money. This neatly sidestepped the humiliating need for any customer to actually have to say the words "sanitary napkin" or "menstruation" out loud.

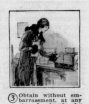

Kotex, Kimberly-Clark, 1920s

1927

After the Lister's Towels debacle, Johnson & Johnson introduced Modess. Modess became Kotex's major competitor in a field of literally hundreds of sanitary pad manufacturers.

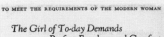

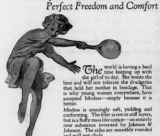

Johnson & Johnson

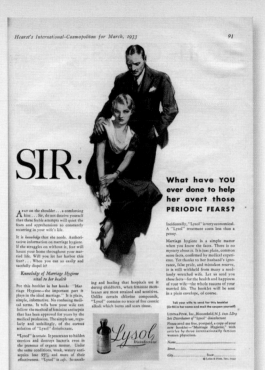

1933

1930–1960

For years, Lysol disinfectant was used as a female contraceptive, as well as a kitchen and bathroom cleanser. Even though it didn't actually prevent pregnancy, ads touted it as "a feminine hygiene product for married women," code for birth control. Testimonials from prominent European "doctors" spoke of its effectiveness, but investigation by the American Medical Association showed that these experts didn't exist and that Lysol didn't kill sperm. But it did kill bathroom germs.

1931

Tampax was born . . . or at least conceived. Dr. Earle Haas filed for a tampon patent—the first to incorporate an applicator, the tube-within-a-tube design that's still used today. After Kotex passed on the patent (much to their subsequent chagrin), Gertrude Tendrich bought it for $32,000 and founded Tampax in 1933. At first she made tampons at home, using a sewing machine and Dr. Haas's compression machine.

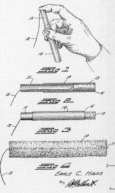

United States Patent Office, 1932

1930s

Lenora Chalmers patented and produced the first reusable menstrual cup. Yet after the advent of disposable products, not many women wanted to handle their blood when they could simply flush or throw it away.

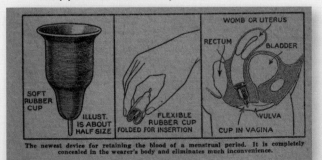

SOFT RUBBER CUP
ILLUST. IS ABOUT HALF SIZE
FLEXIBLE RUBBER CUP FOLDED FOR INSERTION
WOMB OR UTERUS
RECTUM
BLADDER
VULVA
CUP IN VAGINA

The newest device for retaining the blood of a menstrual period. It is completely concealed in the wearer's body and eliminates much inconvenience.

Romantic Confessions magazine, 1934

1950s

Pursettes, a nonapplicator tampon with a lubricated tip, went on sale. Tampon cases were also for sale (separately) so teenage girls—their target audience—could effectively hide tampons in their purses. "Purse." "Pursettes." Cute.

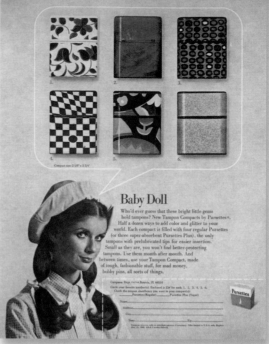

Pursettes, 1968

1948

The "Modess . . . because" print campaign was launched, turning menstrual advertising into a showcase for high-end couture and fashion photography.

1951

While the Catholic Church was adamantly opposed to artificial birth control, Pope Pius XII announced that the Church would sanction the "rhythm method."

1959

Menstrual cups got a second chance when Tassette reintroduced them, this time with a big advertising push. Women still weren't interested, and the cup disappeared again.

Glen Raven Mills invented pantyhose, and overnight, women had a more secure way to help hold pads in place. At least it beat the stockings/garter/sanitary belt combination.

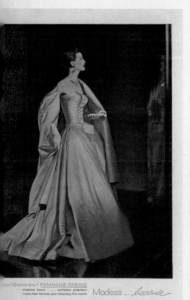

Modess, Johnson & Johnson, 1958

Tassaway, 1971

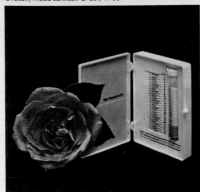

1960

Enovid, the first birth control pill, was approved by the FDA. While the Pill revolutionized contraception and jump-started the sexual revolution, it had dangerous side effects, including life-threatening blood clots and heart attacks. It turns out the dosage was ten times higher than it needed to be. Eleven women died and over a hundred suffered from blood clots, but Searle (Enovid's manufacturer) claimed there was no concrete evidence against the Pill. It took almost ten years to conclusively prove that link.

1968

In *Humanae Vitae* (Of Human Life), Pope Paul VI shared his views on the Pill, saying that it "opened up a wide and easy road . . . toward conjugal infidelity and the general lowering of morality. Man, growing used to contraceptive practices, may lose respect for the woman and come to the point of considering her as a mere instrument of selfish enjoyment, and no longer as his respected and beloved companion." He didn't mention how the woman felt about it.

1963

The Feminine Mystique was published, and Betty Friedan gave a voice to multitudes of discontented housewives across the country.

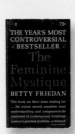

1969

Stayfree minipads, the first sanitary pads with adhesive strips, went on sale, signaling the end of belts, clips, and safety pins for millions of women.

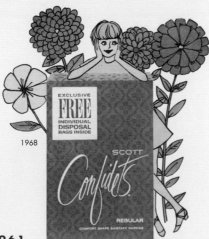

1968

1961

Confidets were the first contoured pads—wider in the front, narrower in the back, for a more comfortable fit. They were also the first to be sold with disposal bags. The brand preferred by American women according to the *Consumer Reports Guide* of 1978, Confidets were discontinued in the 1980s.

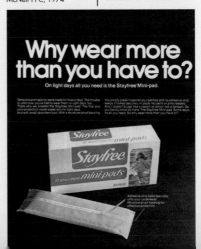

Why wear more than you have to?

On light days all you need is the Stayfree Mini-pad.

1970s

Panty liners became all the rage. While they were initially advertised for light days or for tampon backup, many women were soon wearing them every day.

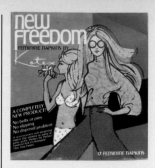

1970

The young adult novel *Are You There God? It's Me, Margaret* was published. For generations, Judy Blume let girls live vicariously through the realities of puberty, preteen angst, first kisses, and first periods.

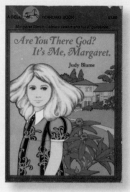

1972

Kimberly-Clark joined the beltless generation with New Freedom pads.

The National Association of Broadcasters lifted its ban on television advertising of sanitary napkins, tampons, and douches.

The U.S. Supreme Court ruled in *Eisenstadt v. Baird* that a state (in this case, Massachusetts) could not prohibit the sale of contraceptives to unmarried women.

1971

Personal Products Company introduced Stayfree maxipads.

Menstrual extraction hit the scene. Lorraine Rothman and Carol Downer toured the country, encouraging women to join self-help groups and extract each other's menses. Amazingly enough, it was immensely popular and over 20,000 procedures were performed. In fact, it wasn't just menstrual blood that was being extracted; embryos, either detected or undetected, were removed, as well. After *Roe v. Wade* made abortion legal in 1973, the popularity of menstrual extractions waned.

In her bestselling book *Living on the Earth*, Alicia Bay Laurel suggested women make tampons by cutting cellulose kitchen sponges into strips, which could be reused after rinsing.

Playtex introduced the first deodorant tampon, a curiosity in itself, seeing that menstrual blood doesn't develop an odor until after it leaves the body.

United States Patent Office, 1974

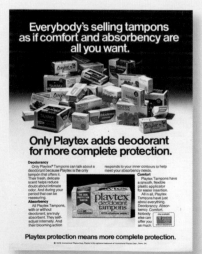

Everybody's selling tampons as if comfort and absorbency are all you want.

Only Playtex adds deodorant for more complete protection.

Deodorancy
Only Playtex® Tampons can talk about a deodorant because Playtex is the only tampon that offers it. Their fresh, delicate scent helps reduce doubt about intimate odor. And during your period that can be reassuring.

Absorbency
All Playtex Tampons, with or without deodorant, are truly absorbent. They self-adjust internally. And their blooming action

responds to your inner contours to help meet your absorbency needs.

Comfort
Playtex Tampons have a smooth, flexible plastic applicator for easier insertion. All in all, Playtex Tampons have just about everything. Deodorancy. Absorbency. Comfort. Nobody else can offer you as much.

Playtex protection means more complete protection.

1974

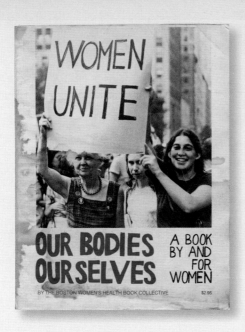

1973

Our Bodies, Ourselves was published. Written for women, by women, it dealt frankly with menstruation, birth control, childbirth, menopause, sexuality, mental health, and many other issues that had been taboo to discuss.

1980

Procter & Gamble took Rely off the market after the tampons were linked to deadly Toxic Shock Syndrome.

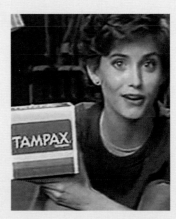

1975

Rely tampons ("we even absorb the worry") went on sale.

Modess patented a flushable sanitary napkin. They may have been flushable, but they also clogged pipes and are no longer for sale.

1985

Courteney Cox Arquette used the word "period" for the first time in a TV commercial.

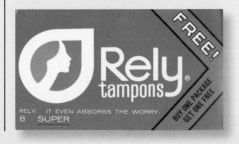

1987

The Keeper, yet another incarnation of the reusable menstrual cup, went on sale. These were somewhat successful and are still on the market.

Late 1980s

The medical profession announced that regular douching was bad for the vagina, altering its pH balance, which could promote infection. Even so, women continue to spend millions of dollars on douching products.

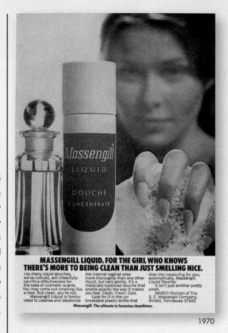

MASSENGILL LIQUID. FOR THE GIRL WHO KNOWS THERE'S MORE TO BEING CLEAN THAN JUST SMELLING NICE.

Too many liquid douches, we've noticed, will cheerfully sacrifice effectiveness for the sake of cosmetic scents. You may come out smelling like a rose. But clean, you're not. Massengill Liquid is formulated to cleanse and deodorize

the internal vaginal area more thoroughly than any other liquid, but very gently. It's a medically balanced douche that smells exactly the way it makes you feel. Clean. Fresh. Cool.
Look for it in the unbreakable plastic bottle that

does the measuring for you, automatically. Massengill Liquid Douche.
It isn't just another pretty smell.

MASCO Division of The S. E. Massengill Company, Bristol, Tennessee 37620

Massengill. The ultimate in feminine cleanliness.

1970

1995

A completely new menstrual product, Fresh 'n' Fit Padettes, went on sale. A super minipad for light days, it was designed to be tucked horizontally between the folds of the labia. Initial studies showed that women were enthusiastic about them, but they soon disappeared.

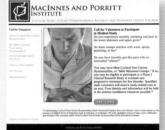

2006

The popular Web site menwith-cramps.com is highlighted on Leno, mentioned in *The New York Times*, and gets 38 million hits. It's revealed to be a parody Web site sponsored by Procter & Gamble to promote ThermaCure HeatWraps, an actual product for menstrual cramps. Apparently, the whole idea of male cramps is a delightful online romp, whereas female cramps, not so much.

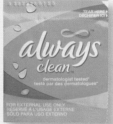

2005

A patent was issued for the Personal Pelvic Viewer, which, according to the company's Web site, "will allow women to choose, by themselves, to take substantial control over their own bodies for the first time in human history" by watching their lady parts on a TV or computer screen.

2007

Always Clean is launched, the first pads packaged with individually wrapped wipes. According to their ads, "Now you can feel shower clean without the shower." You can also subject sensitive tissue to unnecessary chemicals while adding more packaging to landfills.

2003

The FDA approved the first continuous birth control pill, which both suppresses periods and provides birth control. Women taking Seasonale have just four menstrual periods a year.

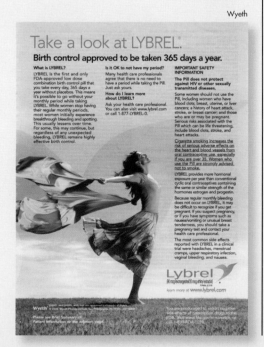

Lybrel is approved by the FDA—the first birth control pill to eliminate periods altogether. That being said, the Web site freely admits that women may experience "menstrual cramps and vaginal bleeding." Hey . . . isn't that actually a period?

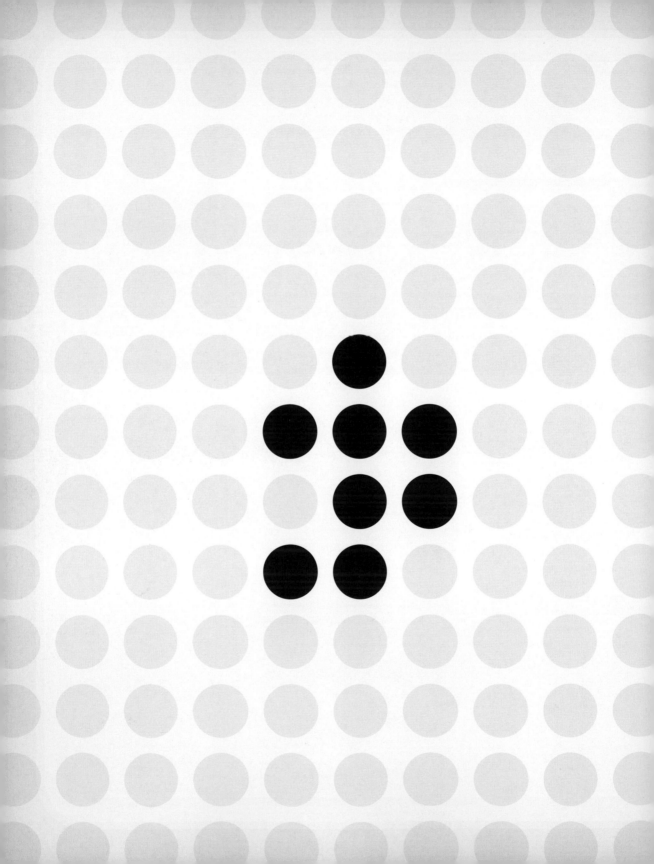

Chapter 8

ADVERTISING

Tampax makes life worth living.
— TAMPAX AD (1939)

HEY, WE WEREN'T BORN YESTERDAY.
We understand that TV commercials aren't teeny, tiny documentaries intended to mirror life. Advertising is meant to sell, first and foremost, and not just a specific brand of tampons, pickles, or life insurance. If it's done right, a good ad also manages to sell emotions, fantasies, fears, and lifestyles.

We understand this, we really do; and yet we also can't help noticing the fact that women are incredibly diverse when it comes to how they experience menstruation. When it comes to our flow, we have a wide range of symptoms, attitudes, problems, and joys, even at different times in our own lives. So why is this never once referred to in femcare ads? Why are the women featured never moody, angry, introspective? Or bloated, or constipated, or covered with a fresh crop of pimples? Or doubled over with cramps, or manic with creative energy? When P&G tells us to "have a happy period. Always," are they being sincere? Or is this the ad-speak

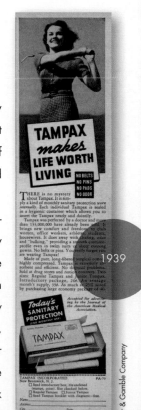

1939

47

version of "have a nice day," in which the point is to end the discussion as fast as possible without being overtly rude? If menstrual advertising doesn't reflect real life in any sense of the word—involving real women, recognizable situations, and actual goo—what does it *do*, anyway?

We're glad you asked, because we've been mulling this over a long time. What we realized femcare ads actually do, and quite efficiently, is rigorously drill us on the constantly evolving vocabulary of new product improvements and development.

If you don't believe us, just think of phrases like "feminine wipe," "pearlescent applicators," and "leak-lock system." Trust us, you weren't born knowing this stuff; after all, if you had mentioned "four-wall protection" or "flexi-wings" back in the 1970s, people would have figured you either owned a construction business or worked for Boeing.

But that's not all that's going on.

Advertisers and manufacturers have also created a shadow code that lurks beneath the vaguely scientific-sounding terminology of absorption technology and applicator design. This secret language consists primarily of friendly, cozy words you'd expect your elderly school nurse to use, like "shower fresh," "confident," "protection," "safe," and "dainty." And yet this code, firmly in place since the dawn of femcare ads, has been instrumental in teaching us a far darker lesson than what "leakage barrier" really means.

To sell their products effectively, femcare ads have successfully tapped into the centuries-old message that the process itself is unspeakable and a source of deep shame. While such ads didn't invent self-loathing, they sure as hell capitalized on it, promulgating a sense of bodily mortification we all should have outgrown decades ago. As a result, advertisers have profoundly influenced what we know and how we think and feel not just about our periods, but our very bodies. Not to be overly dramatic, but one could say our collective menstrual mind-set is the result of effective advertising campaigns.

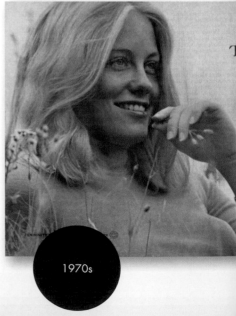

1970s

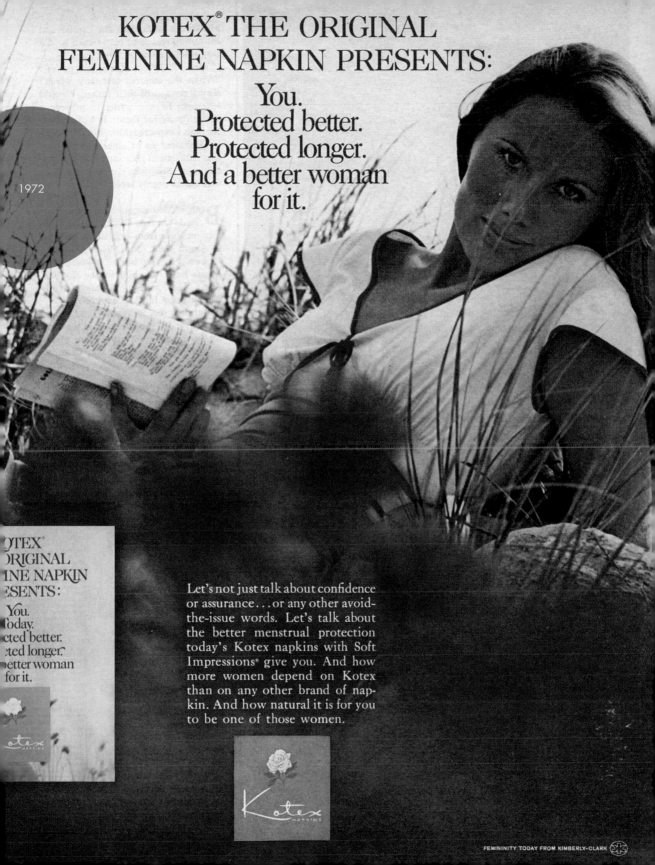

KOTEX® THE ORIGINAL
FEMININE NAPKIN PRESENTS:
You.
Protected better.
Protected longer.
And a better woman
for it.

1972

Let's not just talk about confidence or assurance...or any other avoid-the-issue words. Let's talk about the better menstrual protection today's Kotex napkins with Soft Impressions® give you. And how more women depend on Kotex than on any other brand of napkin. And how natural it is for you to be one of those women.

Kotex
NAPKINS

FEMCARE PROMISES TO KEEP YOUR SECRET

With tampons, girls can feel perfectly confident wearing slacks, shorts, sheaths, or swimsuits. For nothing can show and no one can tell.

—TAMPAX (1966)

Tampons fit into even the smallest of date-size purses, thus making it easy to stay fresh through an evening of fun. When tampons are used, there's not the slightest chance of a telltale outline being visible.

—TAMPAX (1966)

Your narrow Kotex belt won't show under the tightest dress. And neither will your Kotex pad. For Kotex has flat, pressed ends that never make tell-tale outlines . . . never give your secret away.

—KOTEX (1943)

Comfort, and the certainty that our secret's safe, are of the utmost importance to our peace of mind during those "off-days" . . . and it all depends on the type of sanitary protection we use.

—BELTX (1955)

Why tampons? Because tampons are today. They're the "now" product invented to give young women internal menstrual protection. Like today's uninhibiting fashions, tampons give you a new kind of freedom. Invisibility is one of their greatest assets.

—KOTEX (1974)

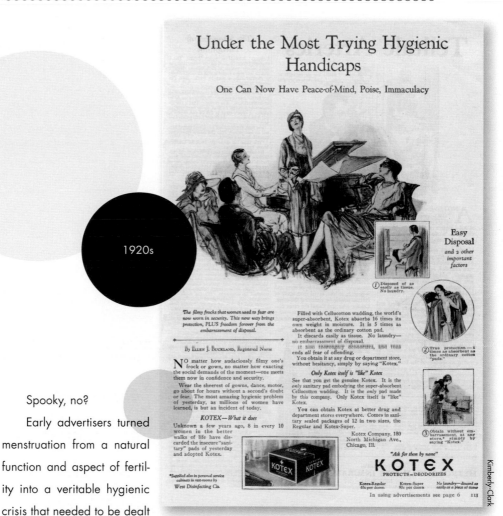

1920s

Spooky, no?

Early advertisers turned menstruation from a natural function and aspect of fertility into a veritable hygienic crisis that needed to be dealt with by the big boys: scientists, the medical community, and last but not least, your trustworthy pad and tampon makers. Fair enough—it was the early twentieth century, manufacturers were trying to scare up business for a new product, and what's more, back then, you could hardly say the word "pregnant" in mixed company without being run out of town on a rail. But what disconcerts us is that the very same tactics that were used nearly a century ago are still very much alive and thriving, and have cumulatively warped our attitudes.

From the very first menstrual ads in the 1920s to the one in this week's *People* (and you can check for yourself if you don't believe us), advertising's double-pronged message has remained eerily constant, albeit with different hairstyles: that (A) menstruation is horrible and embarrassing and God forbid anyone get wise to the fact you're actually bleeding, and (B) their products and theirs alone will bring you boundless protection.

So how did this all get started?

Disposable femcare hit the market, or rather tiptoed timidly in, bringing with it an inherent head-scratcher for its advertisers: how to educate a profoundly repressed market that was horrified enough seeing the bare legs of a sofa, much less those of a woman, about not just any ol' new product, but one that addressed such a personal female function.

The answer came like a bolt from the blue, in what would become one of advertising's core tenets: capitalize on human insecurity. If you can first convince a potential customer that she has a serious problem, then somehow talk her into believing that you, and only you, hold the solution . . . why then, she'll leap on whatever you're selling like white on rice!

The first step—convincing women that menstruation was a problem—turned out to be relatively easy, thanks to the early-1920s obsession with germs and bacteria. If you don't believe us, just consider that the company Listerine actually invented the term "chronic halitosis" in 1921. Implying bad breath was not merely a social problem but a medical one, Listerine went on to make hay (and huge profits) by exploiting that particular anxiety for decades.

If preying on concocted anxiety about bad breath worked so well, why not try it on menstruation? The first Kotex ads ran in 1921 and focused exclusively on hygiene and personal cleanliness.

But the anxieties those early ads preyed on weren't just your garden-variety jitters about hygiene and the possible humiliation of filth. They were also profoundly about money and class.

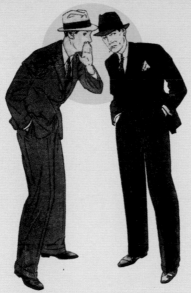

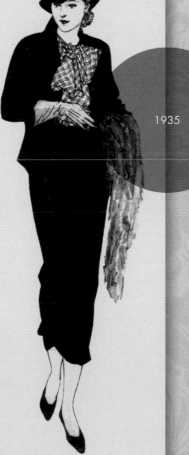

1935

WOMEN
Men Despise

THERE are a [number] of them in every large office. If your luck's bad you often [saw] one as a partner at the bridge table. In [mo]vie theatres they sit next to you—or, what [is worse], back of you. You see them lurking [in] the corner at parties, trying to look as if [th]ey were enjoying themselves. They're [ev]erywhere—these women men despise.

What does it matter that they are attractive [an]d engaging if they commit the offense un[par]donable? Who cares about their beauty and [ch]arm if between stands that insurmountable [hur]dle, halitosis (unpleasant breath).

You Never Know

[Yo]u yourself never know when you have [hali]tosis (unpleasant breath). That's the in[sid]ious thing about it. But others do, and [jud]ge you accordingly.

[Bad] breath affects everyone at some time [or] other. Ninety percent of cases, says one [den]tal authority, are caused by the fermenta[tio]n of tiny food particles that the most care[ful] tooth brushing has failed to remove. As a [res]ult, even careful, fastidious people often offend. And such offenses are unnecessary.

Why Offend Others?

The safe, pleasant, quick precaution against this condition is Listerine, the safe antiseptic and quick deodorant. Simply rinse the mouth with it morning and night and between times before business or social engagements. Listerine instantly combats fermentation and then overcomes the odors it causes.

Is It Worth The Gamble?

When you want to be certain of real deodorant effect, use only Listerine, which deodorizes longer. It is folly to rely on ordinary mouth washes, many of which are completely devoid of deodorant effect. It is well to remember that excessively strong mouth washes are not necessarily better deodorants. Much of Listerine's deodorant effect is due to other properties than its antiseptic action.

Keep Listerine handy in home and office and use it systematically. It is a help in making new friends and keeping old ones. Lambert Pharmacal Company, St. Louis, Missouri.

LISTERINE *checks* halitosis (BAD BREATH) *deodorizes longer*

McNeil-PPC

Above All Things, This Brings You Peace-of-Mind:
Sheerest, gayest gowns; your flimsiest, daintiest things—
wear them without a moment's thought! . . .
Eight in every ten women in the better walks of
life have adopted this new way.

—KOTEX AD (1926)

Think about it. The intended commercial femcare customer, after all, wasn't the impoverished slob of a woman who was accustomed to dealing with her flow for free, if at all, with rags and bits of sheepskin: the factory worker sewing shirtwaists at her sewing machine, the farmwoman toiling in the fields, the faceless maids, cooks, and laundresses. No, sir; early advertisers took shrewd aim at the women who actually had a little cash to burn.

As a result, Kotex ads from the very beginning featured women who represented this ideal market: exquisite, exclusively white, fabulously wealthy ladies of fashion and leisure. This menstrual fantasy lasted for decades: an idealized femcare world of designer frocks, exotic locales, horseback riding, and resorts—all within your trembling grasp, it was implied, *if you only bought their product!*

From the beginning, Kotex promised the world, and while it didn't necessarily deliver, it did in fact dominate the market, sprinting effortlessly ahead of its many competitors for years.

Dr. Lillian Gilbreth was an early pioneer of market research (and, funnily enough, also the subject, along with her husband and twelve kids, of the bestselling novel *Cheaper by the Dozen*, which later mutated unrecognizably into a 2003 Steve Martin movie). She put together perhaps one of the earliest comprehensive studies of

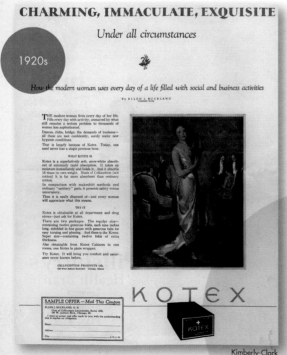

Kimberly-Clark

Kotex is confidence

You'll welcome the newest Kotex napkins. They have a much softer

covering for greater comfort, pleated ends for a smoother fit, also a new inner shield

which provides lasting protection in all 3 absorbencies.

REGULAR   JUNIOR   SUPER

Kimberly-Clark

MOTHER
DON'T BE QUAINT

MILLIONS of daughters are teasing mothers back to youth—slamming doors on the quaint ways of the nineties. One by one the foolish old drudgeries and discomforts pass. Living becomes easier, more pleasant—*sensibly modern*.

An example of this modern trend is Modess. Modess has three vital superiorities—it is really comfortable, can be disposed without danger of clogging and is an effective deodorant.

Its comfort is almost unbelievable, the first time you try it. Modess is graciously soft, yielding, conforming. The filler is not in stiff layers but is a fluffy mass like cotton —an entirely new substance invented by Johnson & Johnson, world's leading makers of surgical dressings.

The sides are smoothly rounded and the specially softened Johnson & Johnson gauze is cushioned with a film of downy cotton.

The deodorizing efficiency of Modess has been proved by laboratory tests to be higher than that of other napkins.

We are sure that you will be delighted to have discovered in Modess a napkin without fault— infinitely more comfortable, safer, more deodorizing and truly disposable. Since it costs no more, why not try it? It may be bought at most good stores.

Johnson & Johnson
NEW BRUNSWICK.   N.J.U.S.A.

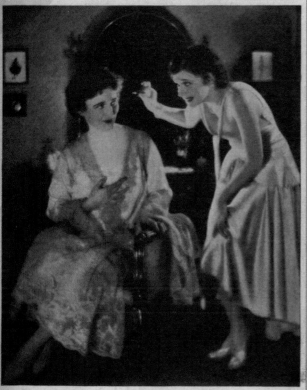

MODERNIZING MOTHER... *Episode Number One*

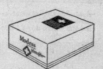

Modess
SO INFINITELY FINER

WOMAN'S WORLD
Remade

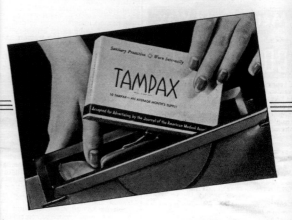

A FEW short months ago many women heard about Tampax for the first time. Since then hundreds of women have written to us to express their gratitude…and to tell us what a difference such a seemingly small detail has made in their lives.

They feel that, for the first time, sanitary protection for the modern woman is adequately solved. For Tampax is worn internally. It is an adaptation of the medical tampon (for internal absorption) perfected for regular monthly use. Of surgical cotton, highly absorbent, compressed, it is easy to use, yet it affords protection that is complete and safe. Gynecologists recommend it as hygienic, civilized and sure. Its advantages are obvious. Belts, pins, pads are, of course, eliminated. In fact, the wearer is completely unconscious of its presence. The ease and freedom made possible by Tampax are unbelievable to the woman who first tries it.

Its other advantages are numerous. Odor is eliminated, because Tampax prevents its formation. Chafing, bulkiness, binding become merely a memory of what soon seems a dark era. Feminine daintiness, ease and comfort are assured at all times.

A month's supply of Tampax comes in a purse-size package. For sale at drug and department stores. 35¢. Instructions for use are included in every package.

TAMPAX Incorporated

IF YOUR LOCAL STORE HAS NOT YET STOCKED TAMPAX
Write to us enclosing 35¢ in stamps or coin and we will gladly mail you a package. Tampax Incorporated, Department C-1, New Brunswick, N. J.
ACCEPTED FOR ADVERTISING BY THE JOURNAL OF THE AMERICAN MEDICAL ASSOCIATION

Procter & Gamble Company

what women *really* felt about femcare and discovered, for starters, that college girls and businesswomen were more likely to buy ready-made supplies than make their own. She also found out that of the fifty-plus brands of commercial femcare currently available, women found almost all of them markedly uncomfortable, especially Kotex. Based on her findings, Modess decided to start from scratch by reinventing the product's image and advertising a different message to a completely new market.

Even though the actual word "teenager" wouldn't even be coined for at least another ten years, early Modess ads egged on generational friction by shamelessly fawning over the youth market it wanted desperately to win over, while simultaneously dumping on their stodgy old mothers:

> *Youth—which will not tolerate senseless drudgery,*
> *the slavery of old-fashioned ways . . .*
> — M O D E S S   A D   (1 9 2 9)

In the early 1930s, the attempt to introduce commercial tampons—plugs of cotton that you were actually supposed to stick up your lady parts!—made the launch of disposable pads look like a stroll through a park. The notion itself was radical, weird, and distinctly off-putting; after all, the act of inserting a tampon conjured up all kinds of unpleasant associations of not only masturbation, but sexual intercourse and even potential defloration . . . eek! As a result, early tampon advertisers took great pains to aim their message exclusively at married women. At the same time, they felt it behooved them not to alienate pad users, either.

> *It's a startling idea, but results are wonderful!*
> — T A M P A X   A D   (1 9 3 0 s)

Another angle tampon advertisers tentatively ran up the flagpole to see if anyone saluted was the recent passage of the Nineteenth Amendment, giving women the right to vote:

All the world is talking of this new emancipation of women.
A new type of sanitary protection, worn internally.

—TAMPAX AD (1930)

But given how leaky those early plugs were, "internal protection" wasn't really what you'd call the tampon's biggest selling point. It was actually what the tampon *didn't* have that gave it any kind of edge at all over the pad: namely belts, pins, and all that shifting, chafing, sweaty bulk. Furthermore, of course, tampons didn't have any of the pad's potential for lingering odor.

In the 1920s and '30s, menstrual odor wasn't just of cosmetic concern, it was linked to a deeper paranoia about germ-ridden, marriage-ending *nastiness*. As a result, there were powerful chemical powders and antiseptics for douching, such as Zonite and Lysol, that preyed on women's darkest, most unspoken anxieties.

In fact, much of early femcare was beset by the kind of quackery you'd expect from such Wild West, preregulatory times. Midol, which originally went on sale in 1911, used to be chock-full of amidopyrine, an anti-inflammatory that could cause agranu-locytosis—a dangerous, even life-threatening condition in which the body's white blood cell count plummets, just like the stock market did in 1929. And up through the mid-1930s, "nostrums," or patent remedies, were touted as a way to cure cramps, heavy periods, unwanted pregnancies, and any uterus in need of toning. Nostrums were wildly popu-

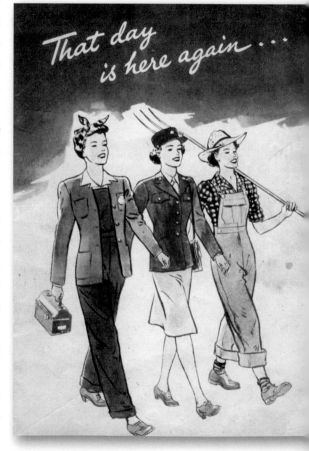

That day is here again . . .

lar, despite not only their hefty price tag but the fact that they were unproven, untested, sometimes dangerous, and often useless.

Funnily enough, the one event that had perhaps the greatest impact on menstrual advertising in history came not from the medical community or even a federal regulatory agency, but from America's entry into World War II.

During the war, women were supposed to contribute to the war effort. Suddenly, they were being urged to buck up, take it on the chin, and above all, not give ol' Mr. Menstrual Discomfort the time of day. "Paying too much attention to it makes about as much sense as listening to your heart beat—or your breathing!" barked one ad, with appropriately drill sergeant–like sternness.

1943

That day is here again!...

Answers for the Woman who asks: "How Can I Feel Better and Stay on the Job *Every* Day of the Month?"

Remember how it was, just a few short years ago —sit around the office, or somebody's bridge table, chattering over clothes and men . . . movies and permanents . . . Mrs. Hoosis's hat?

Seems like a lifetime since then, doesn't it? Since you traded dimity for denim; cocktail frocks for a Service uniform.

Because today, you're a different woman. So busy you can hardly call your soul your own. So *important* that a whole nation's counting on you— to say nothing of that certain Tall Lady With The Torch, standing out in New York harbor.

And now that you're doing a man's job, you're bound you'll see it through (so help you!). To prove to Johnny Doughboy that women "can take it." That *you're* a round-the-month soldier, too.

And then . . . often when you're busiest . . .

Kotex, Kimberly-Clark

Overnight, it became downright treasonous to let one's period stand in the way of efficiency and productivity. What's more, for a brief, shining moment, femcare ads even featured a genuinely egalitarian, classless ideal:

> *Do you belong to one of the groups shown there?*
> *If so, then you really must discover Tampax:*
> *Housewives, war workers, secretaries, students, service workers, sales clerks, gardeners, taxidrivers, club women, teachers, nurses, bank tellers.*
> — TAMPAX AD (1944)

Yet even the most noble-minded ad managed to contain the message that while welding girders with your social inferiors was swell, it sure didn't beat enticing the right guy into marriage once the darn war was over. And glamour was in; lipstick sales in the 1940s were through the roof, perhaps to compensate for all those hours women spent wearing oil-stained overalls, inspecting tank parts.

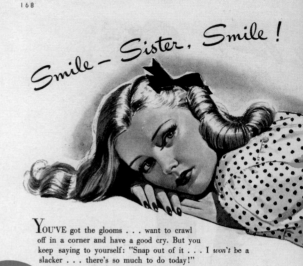

168

Smile — Sister, Smile!

YOU'VE got the glooms . . . want to crawl off in a corner and have a good cry. But you keep saying to yourself: "Snap out of it . . . I *won't* be a slacker . . . there's so much to do today!"

Big important things that mean far more than your own fun and frolics. Things that really matter!

Making bandages this morning. A Defense Stamp luncheon. Then you've simply *got* to finish that navy helmet. And tonight, the boys come home from camp. You'd be a fine citizen spoiling their furlough with a faceful of frowns.

What's the answer? . . . simply give up? NO, a thousand times . . . there *must* be a way to be comfortable and at ease on trying days of the month!

There *is* a way! . . .

Too bad if you're one of those who didn't discover Kotex sanitary napkins long ago! Because if it's comfort you're after . . . you'll find Kotex is *more comfortable!*

For Kotex is made in soft folds so it's naturally less bulky . . . more comfortable . . . made to stay soft while wearing. A lot different from pads that only "feel" soft at first touch.

Kotex does things for your confidence, too . . . builds you up and doesn't let you down! That's because Kotex has flat, pressed ends that keep your secret safe. And a moisture-resistant "safety shield" for *extra* protection.

So try Kotex . . . it won't take you long to discover why it's more popular than all other brands of pads put together. After all, that's *proof* that Kotex stays soft . . . the best proof!

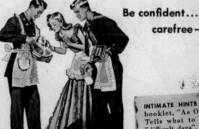

Be confident...comfortable... carefree — with Kotex*!

INTIMATE HINTS FOR GIRLS! New free booklet, "As One Girl To Another" Tells what to do and not to do on "difficult days". Mail name and address to P. O. Box 3434, Dept. M-5, Chicago

(★T. M. Reg. U. S. Pat.

Kimberly-Clark

Early 1940s

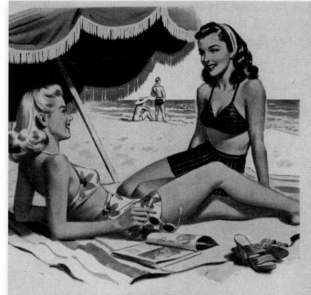

"Meds 'safety-well' gives EXTRA protection!"

No pins, no belts, no revealing "bulges" when you use Meds internal protection! And no worries, either, thanks to the extra security of Meds' exclusive "SAFETY-WELL"!

- Meds are made of real COTTON—soft and super-absorbent for extra comfort.

- Meds alone have the "SAFETY-WELL"—designed for your extra protection.

- Meds' easy-to-use APPLICATORS are dainty, efficient, and disposable.

Meds *only* **20¢**
FOR 10 IN APPLICATORS
Economy package
40 for 65¢!

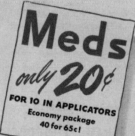

Meds' exclusive "SAFETY-WELL" absorbs so much *more*, so much *faster! Extra* protection for you!
* * *
Meds' fine soft COTTON ca... absorb up to three times its o... weight in moisture! The ... tifically-shaped insorber e... *gently* and *comfortably*—a... itself to individual requi...

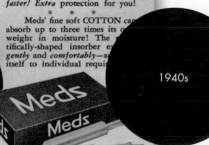

1940s

The 1940s also saw the dawn of sex-goddess advertising. Rita Hayworth, Betty Grable, Veronica Lake—full-length pinups of movie stars were fought over by our boys abroad, and very quickly, super-curvy, glamour-puss models also made their way into our ads at home, advertising everything from shampoo to foot care products to (you guessed it) pads and tampons.

The war ended in 1945 . . . and thanks in large part to the GI Bill and postwar optimism, suburbia was born and the country entered an unprecedented period of prosperity. For once, there was money to spend, as well as some highly skilled ad men telling people how to spend it. Increasingly sophisticated campaigns were created that chose not to sell the specifics of a product, but something more ephemeral and bewitching: the idealized fifties lifestyle.

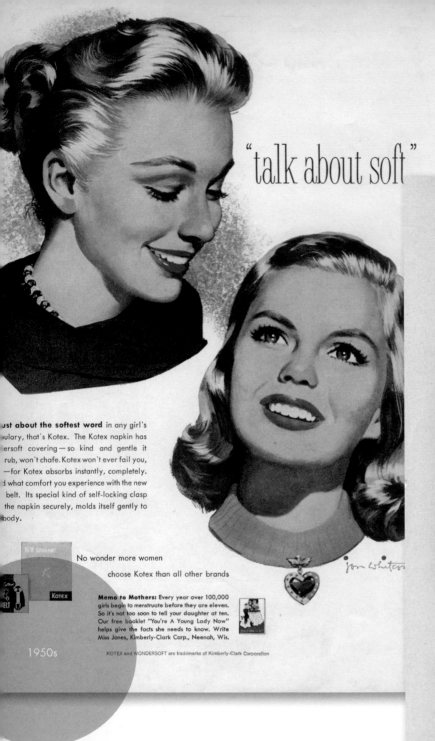

"talk about soft"

...ust about the softest word in any girl's ...ulary, that's Kotex. The Kotex napkin has ...ersoft covering — so kind and gentle it ...rub, won't chafe. Kotex won't ever fail you, ...—for Kotex absorbs instantly, completely. ...d what comfort you experience with the new ... belt. Its special kind of self-locking clasp ... napkin securely, molds itself gently to ...body.

No wonder more women
          choose Kotex than all other brands

Memo to Mothers: Every year over 100,000 girls begin to menstruate before they are eleven. So it's not too soon to tell your daughter at ten. Our free booklet "You're A Young Lady Now" helps give the facts she needs to know. Write Miss Jones, Kimberly-Clark Corp., Neenah, Wis.

1950s

KOTEX and WONDERSOFT are trademarks of Kimberly-Clark Corporation

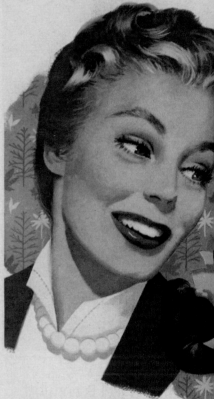

" such gentle so

You'll agree . . . new Kotex napkins are the gentlest ever. For only Kotex has Wondersoft covering . . . so softly spun it won't rub, won't chafe. And you're so sure of yourself with this napkin, for you know it gives you *extra* absorbency that's instant and complete.

For even greater comfort try the new Kotex belt. It's made of woven, non-twist elastic. What's more, it has a special kind of self-locking clasp. This new clasp molds itself comfortably to your body and holds the napkin securely.

No wonder more women
          choose Kotex than all other brands.

KOTEX and WONDERSOFT are trademarks of Kimberly-Clark Corp.

new and
softest ever

New Kotex with Wondersoft covering –the most comfortable, most absorbent napkin ever designed

Now Kotex has Wondersoft covering . . . a new open-mesh covering that's incredibly light and gentle. Only new Kotex napkins with this Wondersoft covering can give you softness you thought you'd never have; complete open-mesh absorption that never fails; and a perfect fit that can't ever pull out of shape.

To complete your comfort, Kotex has created a new sanitary belt. Its soft, flexible clasp ends cutting and chafing . . . yet is actually stronger than metal.

Buy a new
Kotex belt, too!

" . . . a world of difference"

KOTEX and WONDERSOFT are trademarks of Kimberly-Clark Corp.

More women choose KOTEX than all other sanitary napkins

1950s

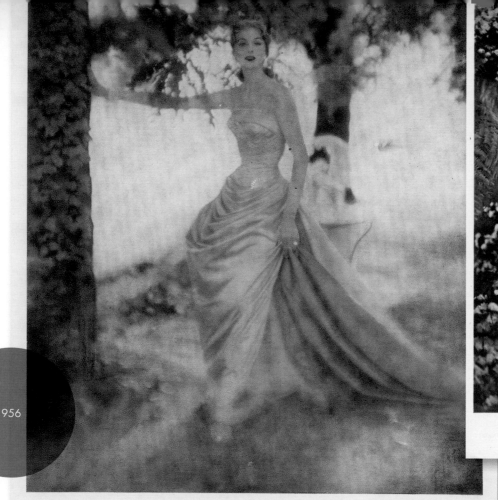

1956

Modess . . . *because*   Only New Design Modess gives you the luxury . . . the gentleness of the fabric covering that's soft as a whisper.

Take, for instance, Young and Rubicam's bizarrely successful "Modess . . . because" campaign for Johnson & Johnson that lasted from 1948 to the 1970s—practically a millennium in advertising years. It created a surreal, virtually wordless world of high fashion, unattainable elegance, and fabulous wealth, with absolutely zero reference to menstruation. Each ad starred undiscovered young beauties like Suzy Parker and Dorian Leigh—effectively launching them into successful careers as the earliest super-models. The ads themselves featured art direction that practically screamed glamour: with couture gowns exclusively designed by Balenciaga, Hattie Carnegie, Valentino, Dior, and all shot by the biggest fashion photographers of the day.

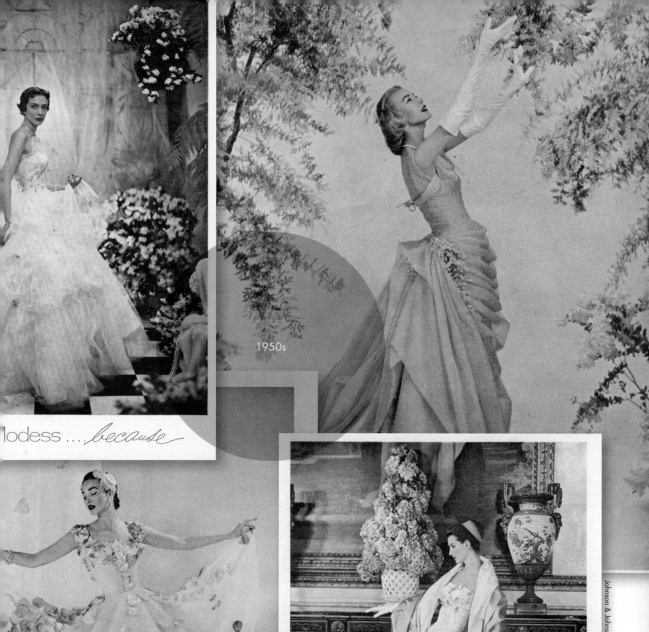

1950s

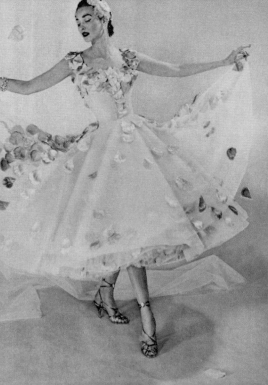

lodess .... *because*

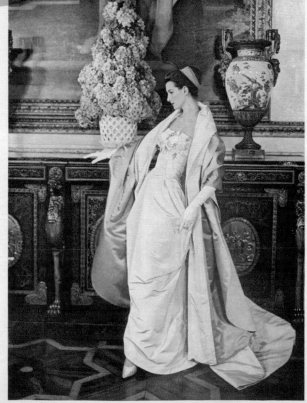

Robert Johnson, of Johnson & Johnson, always said he wanted no more than ten words on any ad. With Modess, he managed to get it down to two: "Modess . . . because." That was it: no explanations, no information, no nothing. The campaign epitomized the new approach to advertising, as sleekly minimalist as an Eames chair, in which less was definitely more. Instead of facts, the ads successfully sold an idealized dream. Moreover, they pitched a new kind of freedom—not social freedom, or physical freedom, or even freedom from those two menstrual standbys, fear and anxiety—but freedom from reality. No wonder the campaign sold a zillion pads!

By the mid-1950s, the new medium called television was exploding and quickly became the obvious, most effective way to advertise. However, femcare had to chill its heels for another fifteen years or so; the National Association of Broadcasters banned advertising of all sanitary napkins, tampons, and douches on TV until 1972.

Nevertheless, femcare print ads continued to flourish in the 1960s, continuing the feel-happy/look-rich trend of the previous decade and violently shying away from anything even vaguely off-putting: product shots, lengthy explanations, anything remotely clinical. What's more, the models in the ads quickly aged down . . . way, *wayyy* down. Hey, it was the Swingin' Sixties, baby! Who wanted to look at some old bag pushing thirty? Older models fell by the wayside like so much cut wood. Overwhelmingly, ads began featuring cute girls bopping around under the sun or gussying up in their fancy frocks: none older than twenty-two, none overweight (or even normal weight), none in dark clothes. And ethnically, all were as white as a Mormon family picnic.

In the 1960s, there wasn't a whisper of racial diversity in menstrual advertising, although to be honest, there wasn't much going on in advertising anywhere, unless one counted commercials for the new Diahann Carroll TV sitcom, *Julia*. In fact, flipping through menstrual ads of the 1960s, one would have nary a clue one was actually in the same era as the civil rights movement, César Chávez, Martin Luther King Jr., and Black Pride.

Menstrual ads from the sixties may not have had much in the way of multiculturalism, but what they *did* have was water: lots and lots of it. Weirdly enough, women were all too frequently depicted sailing, swimming, lounging by the pool, splashing in the surf, flying kites in the surf, building sandcastles, riding horses along the shore, all while ostensibly bleeding merrily away. And what's up with that, you might rightfully wonder?

You don't have to be a Freudian to appreciate that what really comes across from such imagery is the perceived dirtiness of menstruation. In purely visual terms, the message is loud and clear: *all* women need to be ritually cleaned and sanitized after their periods, as if by religious immersion in purifying water.

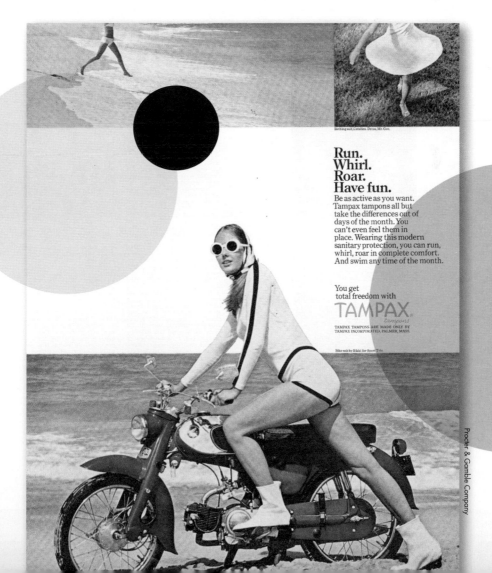

1960s

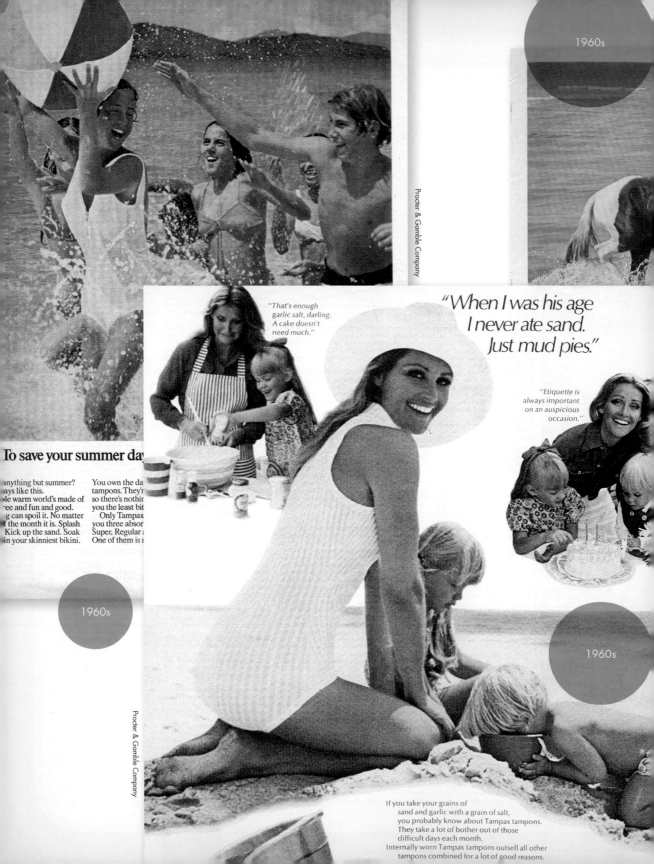

1960s

"That's enough garlic salt, darling. A cake doesn't need much."

"When I was his age I never ate sand. Just mud pies."

"Etiquette is always important on an auspicious occasion."

To save your summer day

anything but summer?
ays like this.
le warm world's made of
ee and fun and good.
g can spoil it. No matter
f the month it is. Splash
Kick up the sand. Soak
in your skinniest bikini.

You own the da
tampons. They'r
so there's nothin
you the least bit

Only Tampax
you three absor
Super, Regular a
One of them is r

1960s

1960s

If you take your grains of
sand and garlic with a grain of salt,
you probably know about Tampax tampons.
They take a lot of bother out of those
difficult days each month.
Internally worn Tampax tampons outsell all other
tampons combined for a lot of good reasons.

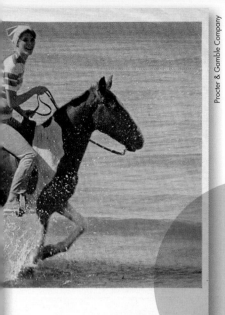

1960s

Make this your summer to remember

Your laughs seem to linger on sea waves, roll out to deep blue water and echo in the calls of distant ships. That's the way summer should always be: that's the way you'll always remember it. Laughter, games, fun. And you're always a part of it when you depend on the internal protection of Tampax tampons. To so many girls, Tampax tampons are a natural part of life. They make even difficult days of summer a time to soak up a golden tan in skinny bikinis, to romp and leap and splash with all your energy. Tampax tampons' internal protection gives you all this freedom and confidence as well.

As the crowd grows and the laughter rises, your worries are a million miles inland. Tampax tampons will protect you dependably. So you can really celebrate a summer to remember.

The internal protection more women trust TAMPAX
tampons

MADE ONLY BY
CANADIAN TAMPAX CORPORATION LTD., BARRIE, ONTARIO

ol, clean, fresh day

You can
de or swim,
s any time of the month.
l cool, clean, fresh
dance all night.
g hampers you,
holds you back
when you use
pax tampons.
et total comfort,
tal freedom.
the least you deserve?

MPAX. modern sanitary protection
tampons
DIAN TAMPAX CORPORATION LTD., BARRIE, ONTARIO.

ly as much
ne beach a

1960s

"I think I'm about to make a big splash."

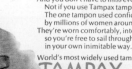

Each day is a new adventure
in this world of watery wonderlands.
And you don't have to miss even a minute.
Not if you use Tampax tampons.
The one tampon used confidently
by millions of women around the world.
They're worn comfortably, internally
so you're free to sail through any day
in your own inimitable way.

World's most widely used tampons...

TAMPAX
tampons
MADE ONLY BY CANADIAN TAMPAX CORPORATION LTD., BARRIE, ONTARIO

"My sunfish solo

But developments in femcare technology, as well as the "second wave" of the women's movement in the late 1960s and early 1970s, seriously knocked off some of the dust mouldering in ad content:

> *Welcome to the beltless, pinless,*
> *fussless generation!*
>
> — NEW FREEDOM AD (1973)

It wasn't just the adhesive strips that made for such a revolution. After decades of elliptical and minimalist ad copy and vague fashion shots, advertisers returned to the role of educator, featuring actual product shots and using descriptive copy in frank (or at least relatively frank) language about exactly what was being sold.

This, of course, was only the case in print ads. The ban on femcare advertising on TV was finally lifted in 1972, and from the ensuing ruckus, you would have thought the networks had started airing live acts of bestiality. Shown only during the women's ghetto of daytime programming blocks, menstrual product commercials

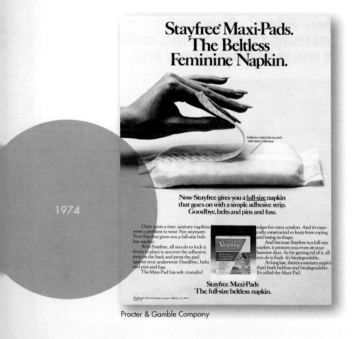

Procter & Gamble Company

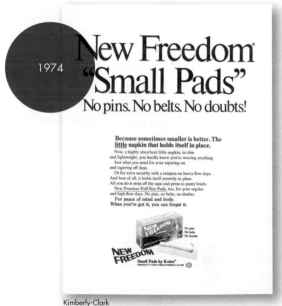

Kimberly-Clark

were instantly met with a thundering roar of unanimous disapproval. It was one thing to flip past an ad in a magazine . . . but on television, right there in front of you? Miss and Mrs. Middle America, apparently, found the whole subject queasy-making, inappropriate, and absolutely the last thing they wanted to see when they were trying to watch *Days of Our Lives* over a nice cup of Sanka. Many manufacturers bravely held off on taking action—that is, until they saw a drop in profits. After that, they beat a hasty retreat back to the tried-and-true code of euphemisms, buzzwords, and soft images. Femcare absorption was soon routinely depicted on TV in a completely bloodless, clinical setting, with menstrual flow represented by sterile blue liquid in a beaker. How much more backpedaling could advertisers do?

Think we're exaggerating? The first time the word "period" was ever used in a TV commercial for tampons wasn't until 1985. Spoken by Courteney Cox Arquette, that one word, part of a national Tampax campaign, unleashed a veritable tsunami of angry letters from outraged viewers across the country. *For Pete's sake . . . what if a child had been in the room? Or God forbid . . . an actual man?*

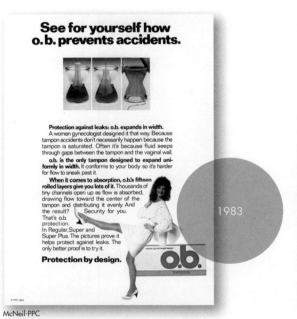

1983

McNeil-PPC

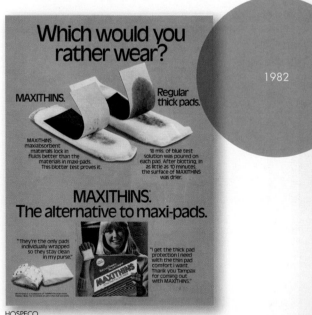

1982

HOSPECO

In our opinion, perhaps the most horrifying femcare ad (albeit for different reasons) was one that aired widely, just a few years earlier:

Rely. It even absorbs the worry.

— RELY AD (1980)

Procter & Gamble's Rely was one of the new breed of superabsorbent tampons launched in the mid-1970s. Tragically, Rely absorbed far more than the worry; it also leached moisture and healthy, natural stuff from the vagina, bringing about a mini-epidemic of Toxic Shock Syndrome. Rely was pulled from the market in 1980 as a sort of whipping boy for the entire tampon industry, since it was clear that the fault lay with the combination of materials used in many, if not most, superabsorbent tampons of the time. Understandably, those were pretty dark days for tampon manufacturers (not to mention for the hundreds of innocent women and girls who were either maimed or killed).

1970s

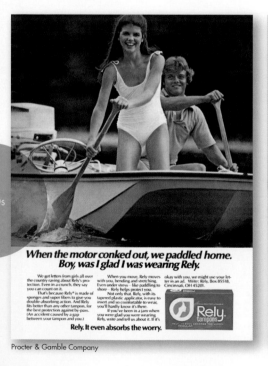

1985

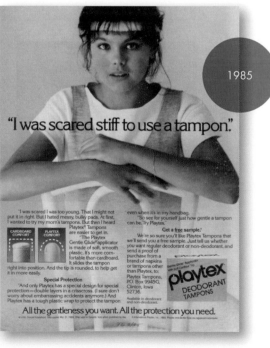

Procter & Gamble Company

Still, after a suitable period of contrition had passed, tampon makers decided that enough was enough, and it was time to get back in the game. And so they mounted a major offensive that was as much anti-pad as it was pro-tampon:

> *I hate pads. They're like wearing diapers.*
>
> — TAMPAX AD (1989)

> *No, the tampon can't get lost. All you can lose are those diapers.*
>
> — TAMPAX AD (1988)

Gone were those innocent days when tampons were marketed at married women only, out of fear of mass deflowerings of virgins. By the 1980s, entire tampon campaigns were aimed squarely at teens . . . and why not? 99.9 percent of all teenage girls live in constant terror of embarrassment, anyway: the fear of leaking, of showing, of being caught holding or buying a femcare product.

> *Gone were those innocent days when tampons were marketed at married women only, out of fear of mass deflowerings of virgins.*

Pad manufacturers, stung to the quick, struck back with all the weapons in their arsenal: citing not only their product's superior safety record when it came to toxic shock, but also its increased absorbency, extra protection, and versatility. After all, pads came as minis, regular, maxis. One could even buy newfangled panty shields, so one could have "extra protection" every day of the month.

The famous Stayfree campaign from the 1980s featured Olympic gymnast Cathy Rigby. Clad in a skin-tight, cleft-revealing leotard, her blond hair in a pert ponytail, Rigby

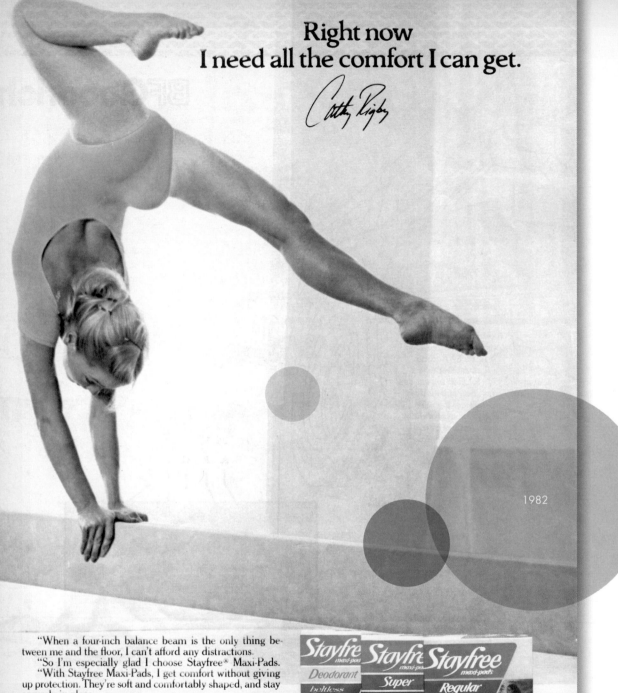

Right now
I need all the comfort I can get.

Cathy Rigby

1982

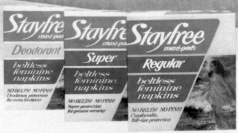

"When a four-inch balance beam is the only thing between me and the floor, I can't afford any distractions.

"So I'm especially glad I choose Stayfree® Maxi-Pads.

"With Stayfree Maxi-Pads, I get comfort without giving up protection. They're soft and comfortably shaped, and stay securely in place.

"So they bend with me, turn with me and never distract me. Stayfree Maxi-Pads are comfort without compromise."

Stayfree® Maxi-Pads.
Comfort without compromise.

STAYFREE is the trademark of **P** *Personal Products Company*, Milltown, N.J. 08850   © PPC 1982 was always shown in extremis: performing splits, leaping about on a balance beam, practically performing a handstand on one pinky. The ads claimed this was all while she was sporting a maxipad, demonstrating that either Stayfree maxipads were as invisible as they claimed to be or someone in the art department was one talented airbrusher.

Cathy Rigby was one of the lucky celebrities who appeared in femcare ads with full knowledge of what she was getting into. Decades earlier, legendary photographer and Surrealist art muse Lee Miller was horrified to find that Kotex had purchased a stock photo of her taken by Edward Steichen and fashioned an ad around her, the first

> *Gymnast Mary Lou Retton and actress Brenda Vaccaro may have hawked tampons, but were made merciless fun of on comedy shows of the day.*

to feature a real person. And while many celebrities throughout history have apparently had few qualms about endorsing cigarettes, booze, gambling, or wearing the fur of endangered animals, getting one to actually plug a plug, so to speak, is a rare event. Fellow gymnast Mary Lou Retton and actress Brenda Vaccaro may have hawked tampons, but were made merciless fun of on comedy shows of the day.

The Internet is now an everpresent marketing and advertising outlet for femcare companies. Every major brand now has an ornate Web site full of peppy photos, womanly advice, serious-sounding information, and above all, an underlying sales pitch.

Tampax has a separate Web site for teenagers, full of girlish talk about slumber parties, underwire bras, boys, and (you guessed it) tampons. Even we have to grudgingly admit that their Web site is kind of, well, *fun*: you can print your own tattoos or head to your dorm room at Tampax U, where you can try on outfits, play with your puppy, and send away for free samples.

At its Web site for teens, Kotex features games, an "attitude explorer" quiz, and message boards, and lets you customize your screen to flower-riffic, groovy green, blue dazzle, or jump 'n' roll. The Always Web site lets you create a cyber Zen garden, download recipes for "spoil me choc chip scones" and "caramel nut popcorn delight," and print out iron-ons for T-shirts. The line between entertainment and advertising is so blurred, there doesn't appear to be one anymore.

> *What do you get for the pad that*
> *has everything?*
> — A L W A Y S   C L E A N   A D   (2 0 0 7)

The past two decades have seen new and improved products, with countless items introduced and hawked. Pads with wings. Sanitary wipes. Pearl tampon applicators— a never-ending parade of shapes and sizes. What's more, femcare companies have also embraced a more positive view of menstruation, even going so far as to encourage women

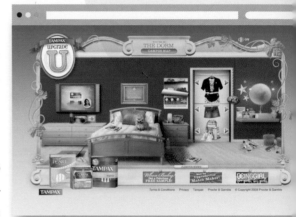

Procter & Gamble Comp

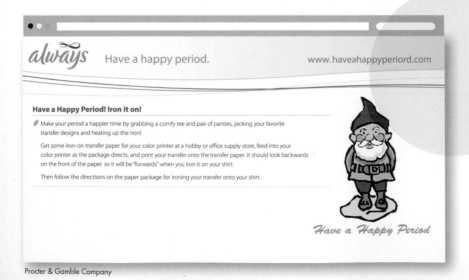

to use their periods as a time for personal indulgence. Yet for all the apparent improvements in both attitude and product development, one disturbing message stays the same: your period is still a secret that should be kept hidden at all costs. By reinforcing this secrecy and the shame that comes with it, menstrual advertising still hasn't changed one bit after all these years.

This is the time of the month that *chocolate* was created for.

This is the time when *no toe nail* should go *unpolished.*

When *going to the mall* is enough of a work out, thank you very much.

This is the time when, if something is even slightly annoying, the *world* should know about it.

And if you *feel* like crying, there is no inappropriate time or place.

It's your period.

You have the right to make it the *best period it can possibly be.* And we're here to help.

Have a happy period. always.

Procter & Gamble Company

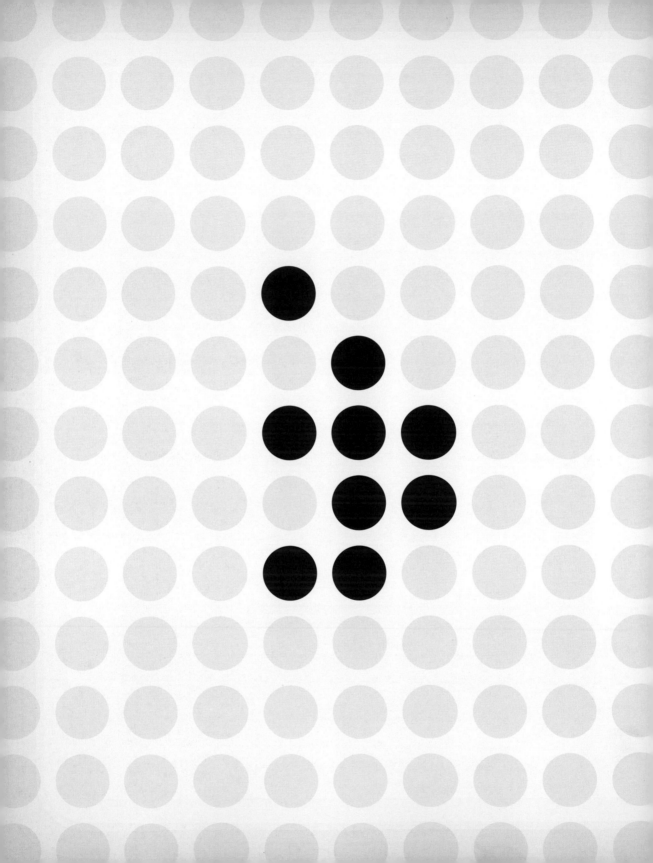

Chapter 9

THE SCENT OF
A WOMAN

ONE QUESTION HAS BEEN SERIOUSLY NAGGING us lately: Does having your period make you smell bad?

An insanely successful industry has built its mighty foundation on the notion that it does—that the odor is not only appalling and disgusting, but that it must be hunted down and destroyed before it eats away your marriage, your standing in society, your very happiness. Just think of the convictions that may very well be lurking in your own brain this very moment about That Smell: that of course menstrual blood stinks, it's been sitting around in your uterus for a whole month getting funky! That if you get your period while you're camping or swimming, bears and sharks will smell you from miles away and immediately come rushing over to eat you! That any civilized male within ten feet will take one sniff of your padded crotch and run for the hills!

And what about the poor old vagina?

Everyone—raise your hand if you've had it up to here with those incredibly stupid and unfunny jokes we've been hearing since junior high about how bad the vagina smells. Unless there's something clinically wrong going on down there, do you honestly think you smell like an old mackerel? Or leftover mussels? Or last week's seafood special at Harry's Clam Shack?

Nevertheless, the vagina itself has very successfully been treated in advertising as not unlike a kitchen counter, bathtub, or worse: i.e., as a foul, germ-ridden receptacle that needs to be vigilantly cleaned, disinfected, and deodorized before one can even think of having company over. Compare this to one's nose, where horrifying viruses often *do* lurk. You wouldn't think of disinfecting the inside of your nose every time you blew it, would you?

A healthy vagina is, in fact, like the rest of the body—a bustling metropolis full of living microorganisms, most of them friendly, a few not so friendly, all coexisting in relative harmony until something occasionally throws the balance off. You could practically hear businessmen rubbing their hands with glee when they hit on the idea of rebranding this normal state of affairs as a problem that women didn't realize they had. The vagina, they declared, was in fact not a happy village, but instead, an undesirable ghetto, a breeding ground for germs and disease . . . *and it needed to be cleaned up!*

> *Superficial or apparent cleanliness has become insufficient for the*
> *modern woman. The discoveries in the fields of medicine, chemistry*
> *and bacteriology have meant a great deal to the health and beauty*
> *of womanhood. . . . The vaginal douche . . . is now universally recom-*
> *mended as an indispensable part of modern woman's toilette . . . !*
>
> —ZONITE AD (1925)

In fact, women may well have been splashing water up into themselves since the days of Cleopatra, but the water they used back then wasn't laced with powerful disinfectants. And what *was* Zonite, anyway? Sphinx-like, all the advertisers would say was that it was "a colorless liquid that destroys odors and leaves no lasting odor of its own. . . . In the presence of the natural secretions of the vaginal tract, it has a greater germicidal power than pure carbolic acid." They added, somewhat ominously, that it could permanently damage clothing, as well.

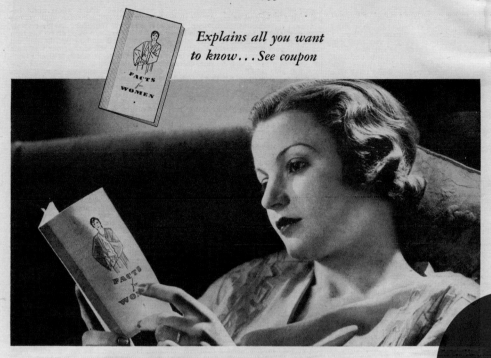

HOW CAN IT BE TACTFULLY TOLD
to a sensitive young wife?

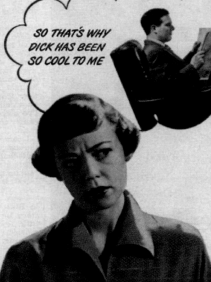

YOU SEE, DEAR, THERE'S A GRAVE WOMANLY OFFENSE THAT'S RARELY DISCUSSED

SO THAT'S WHY DICK HAS BEEN SO COOL TO ME

1930s

No other type liquid antiseptic-germicide tested for the douche is so powerful yet safe to tissues

In this modern age, a woman must realize how wise it always is to put ZONITE in her fountain syringe for hygiene (*internal* cleanliness), for her health, charm, after her periods—and *especially* to follow this hygienic practice when she is married. She must realize there's a very common odor which she herself may not detect but is so apparent to people around her.

AND ISN'T IT REASSURING FOR A WIFE TO KNOW THAT NO OTHER TYPE LIQUID ANTISEPTIC-GERMICIDE TESTED FOR THIS PURPOSE IS SO POWERFULLY EFFECTIVE YET SAFE TO TISSUES AS ZONITE.

Truly a Modern Miracle!

Modern women no longer have to use dangerous products, overstrong solutions of which may gradually cause serious damage. Nor will they want to rely on weak homemade solutions—

© 1950 Z.P.C.

none of which have ZONITE's remarkable deodorizing, germ-killing action.

Developed by a famous surgeon and scientist—this ZONITE principle is POWERFULLY EFFECTIVE YET POSITIVELY NON-POISONOUS, NON-IRRITATING. You can use it as directed as often as you want, without the slightest risk of injury.

Gives BOTH Internal and External Hygienic Protection

ZONITE deodorizes not by just "masking"—it actually destroys, dissolves and removes odor-causing waste substances. Use ZONITE and be assured you won't offend. ZONITE has such a soothing effect and promptly helps relieve itching and irritation if present. ZONITE gives daily *external* hygienic protection, too, leaving you with such a refreshed dainty feeling. Buy ZONITE today!

FREE! NEW!

For amazing enlightening NEW Booklet containing frank discussion of intimate physical facts, recently published—mail this coupon to Zonite Products Corp., Dept. MR-60, 100 Park Avenue, New York 17, N. Y.*

Zonite
FOR NEWER
feminine hygiene

Name_____

Address_____

City_____ State_____

*Offer good only in the U. S.

According to the directions, administering Zonite entailed having to somehow lie underneath eight feet of tubing in one's bathtub, legs propped up and splayed open like a Thanksgiving turkey, as the recommended two quarts of fluid slowly dribbled downward and up into one's unsuspecting vagina. If one wanted to attempt this during one's period, there were even special directions to teach a woman how to deal with those "annoying clots and crustations."

And if that didn't make you want to immediately rush out and buy some, the ad went on to point out that Zonite could also be used to clean wounds, to treat sunburn, eczema, poison ivy, and dandruff, and as a mouthwash and underarm deodorant. That's because Zonite was actually sodium hypochlorite—basically, weak bleach. So why didn't the manufacturer just come right out and say so? Why the big mystery?

This had much to do with the loosey-goosey approach the government used to take in regulating the manufacture and advertising of drugs and medicine. Attempts had been made earlier in the twentieth century to prevent "filthy, decomposed, or putrid" substances from making their way into one's canned ham or bottle of celery tonic. Still, federal laws against drug makers not listing their ingredients (which often included things like opium, cocaine, poison, and various radioactive substances) and making truly nutty claims wouldn't kick in until the late 1930s . . . and this was only after a new, raspberry-flavored elixir meant to kill streptococcal infections actually killed people instead, due to a poisonous ingredient.

As a result, early advertisers in the feminine hygiene business had no qualms about throwing the net wide with their promises. If no one was going to call you out on your wacky claims, much less nail you on a class-action suit, why not promise the moon? Check out this 1935 advertising booklet for yet another douche: "We all know women whose once pink-and-white complexions have turned to a hard sallowness; who have faded from blooming youth to premature middle age; whose skins are rough, pimply, blotched; who tire too easily; who constantly complain of backaches, headaches and other pains; whose body odors are offensive. Feminine hygiene is indicated as the first corrective of these too customary troubles to which nearly 85 out of every 100 women fall prey."

Douching was also touted as being good for "congestion in the pelvic region" and the "accumulation of inactive blood in the womb." And though they might have been accused of gilding the lily, the makers of Certane even thoughtfully bundled up their tubing and nozzles into an attractive gift set.

Even after the FDA finally decided to grow a pair when it came to policing outright charlatanism, douching still continued to be aggressively promoted as the cure for any and all marital ills. After all, wrote Joseph M. Lee sadly in his 1953 book about feminine hygiene, "it is difficult to love that which offends." In one particularly lurid ad from the 1950s, a distraught housewife pleads, "Please, Dave . . . please don't let me be locked out from you!" as she hammers impotently on a closed door festooned with locks and chains labeled "doubt," "inhibitions," and "ignorance." The ad goes on to chide her thusly: "Often a wife fails to realize that doubts due to one intimate neglect shut her out from a happily married love." Get the hint? She stinks to high heaven, and that's why she drove poor Dave away! But the real kicker of this ad isn't just that it's for any old douche . . . it's for (wait for it) *Lysol.*

Yes, we kid you not. Lysol . . . that neon-yellow disinfectant that was scary enough when your mom scrubbed out the toilet bowl with it, and which is still strong enough to

WOMEN'S SECRETS

The Last Word in Feminine Fastidiousness

1935

Certane Ideal Combination Set

This complete vaginal cleansing and feminine hygiene set is one of the most popular among women, and makes an ideal gift.

It contains—
    One tube of Certane Jelly and Applicator (approximately 30 applications). (Or Certane Cones if you prefer.)
    One 12-oz. package Certane Douche Powder
    One Certane Health Shield & Rubber Tubing
Specially Reduced for a Limited Time.................$3.95
(Former price, $7.50). *In convenient box.*
Ideal Combination Set with Dia-Cap or
    Dia-Dome $5.95

[18]

VAGINAL ODOR AS SOAP OPERA

Often a wife fails to realize that doubts due to one intimate neglect shut her out from happy married love. **—LYSOL**

Before long this sense of misgiving developed into nervous irritability. Slowly but surely I could see the man I loved turning from me. **—ZONITE**

Day after heartbreaking day I was held in an unyielding web . . . a web spun by my husband's indifference. **—LYSOL**

A marriage may sometimes lose all the glorious magic of romance . . . even wreck completely . . . because of a wife's carelessness (or ignorance) about Feminine Hygiene. It could happen to YOU. You surely don't want to risk such a deeply personal tragedy. **—LYSOL**

So humiliated when she realized the cause of her husband's frigidity. **—ZONITE**

kill the Ebola virus without batting an eye. In fact, the very potency of Lysol was considered one of its selling points as a vaginal rinse.

Back then, women understood the veiled hints when ads for Lysol coyly mentioned it was for "married women," for "morning-after freshness." In other words, their product wouldn't simply make your vagina all fresh and dewy-smelling . . . it would also kill any pesky sperm (which were considered pretty close to germs themselves) that might be lurking around up there, as well. This was, after all, also the era when girls not only wore

"PLEASE, DAVE..PLEASE DON'T LET ME BE LOCKED OUT FROM YOU!"

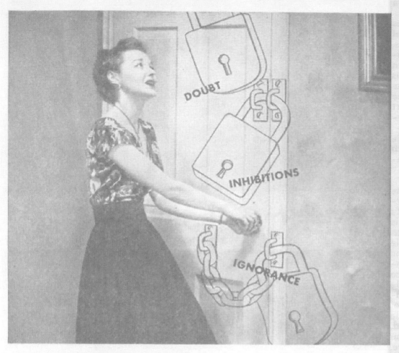

DOUBT

INHIBITIONS

IGNORANCE

Often a wife fails to realize that doubts due to one intimate neglect shut her out from happy married love

A man marries a woman because he loves her. So instead of blaming him if married love begins to cool, she should question herself. Is she truly trying to keep her husband and herself eager, happy married lovers? One most effective way to safeguard her dainty feminine allure is by practicing *complete feminine hygiene* as provided by vaginal douches with a *scientifically correct* preparation like "Lysol." *So* easy a way to banish the misgivings that often keep married lovers *apart*.

Germs destroyed swiftly

"Lysol" has amazing, *proved* power to kill germ-life on contact . . . truly cleanses the vaginal canal even in the presence of mucous matter. Thus "Lysol" *acts* in a way that makeshifts like soap, salt or soda *never can.*

Appealing daintiness is assured, because the very source of objectionable odors is eliminated.

Use whenever needed!

Yet gentle, non-caustic "Lysol" *will not harm* delicate tissue. Simple directions give correct douching solution. Many doctors advise their patients to douche regularly with "Lysol" brand disinfectant, just to insure feminine daintiness alone, and to use it as often as necessary. No greasy aftereffect.

For feminine hygiene, three times more women use "Lysol" than any other liquid preparation. No other is more reliable. You, too, can rely on "Lysol" to help protect your married happiness . . . keep you desirable!

For complete Feminine Hygiene rely on . . .

"*Lysol*"
Brand Disinfectant

A Concentrated Germ-Killer

Product of Lehn & Fink

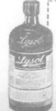

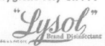

DOUBT

INHIBITION

IGNORANCE

MISGIVINGS

For complete Feminine Hygiene rely on . . .

"*Lysol*"
Brand Disinfectant

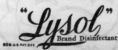

TOO LATE TO CRY OUT IN ANGUISH!

Beware of the one intimate neglect that can engulf you in marital grief

TOO LATE, when love has gone, for a wife to plead that no one warned her of danger. Because a wise, considerate wife makes it her business to *find out* how to safeguard her daintiness in order to protect precious married love and happiness.

One of the soundest ways for a wife to keep married love in bloom is to achieve dainty allure by practicing *effective* feminine hygiene such as *regular* vaginal douches with reliable "Lysol."

Germs destroyed swiftly

"Lysol" has amazing, *proved* power to kill germ-life on contact . . . truly cleanses the vaginal canal even in the presence of mucous matter. Thus "Lysol" *acts* in a way that makeshifts like soap, salt or soda *never can.*

Appealing daintiness is assured, because the very source of objectionable odors is eliminated.

Use whenever needed!

Gentle, non-caustic "Lysol" will not harm delicate tissue. Easy directions give correct douching solution. Many doctors advise their patients to douche regularly with "Lysol" brand disinfectant, just to insure daintiness alone, and to use it as often as they need it. No greasy aftereffect.

For feminine hygiene, three times more women use "Lysol" than any other liquid preparation. No other is more reliable. You, too, can rely on "Lysol" to help protect your married happiness . . . keep you desirable!

- -

V!...FEMININE HYGIENE FACTS!

FREE! New booklet of information by ing gynecological authority. Mail on to Lehn & Fink, 192 Bloomfield ue, Bloomfield, N. J.

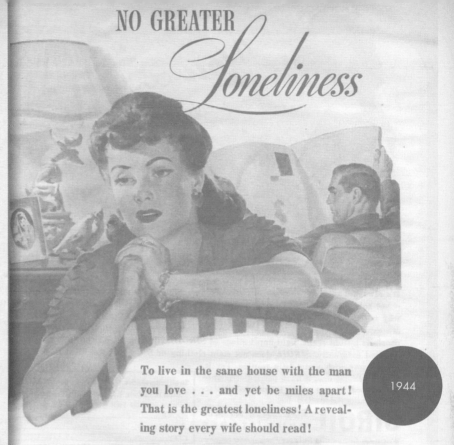

NO GREATER *Loneliness*

1944

To live in the same house with the man you love . . . and yet be miles apart! That is the greatest loneliness! A revealing story every wife should read!

THE silence in the living room was so deep that the ticking of the small desk clock sounded loud and sharp . . . the way it does in the middle of a sleepless night. That—and the rustle of Rod's newspaper were the only sounds in the room since dinner.

Bitterly, Enid remembered the happy evenings they once had shared. Now they shared nothing but the same roof . . . What had come between them?

DOCTORS KNOW that too many women still do not have up-to-date information about certain physical facts. And too many, who think they know, have only half-knowledge. So they still rely on ineffective or dangerous preparations.

You have a right to know about the important medical advances made during recent years in connection with this intimate problem. They affect every woman's health and happiness.

And so, with the cooperation of doctors who specialize in women's medical problems, the makers of Zonite have just published an authoritative new book, which clearly explains the facts. *(See free book offer below.)*

You SHOULD, however, be warned here about two definite threats to happiness. First, *the danger of infection present every day in every woman's life.* Second, *the most serious deodorization problem any woman has* . . . one which you may not suspect. And what to use is so important. That's why you ought to know about Zonite Antiseptic.

USED IN THE DOUCHE (as well as for a simple every-day routine of external protection) Zonite is both antiseptic and deodorant. Zonite deodorizes, not by just masking, but by actually destroying odors. Leaves no lasting odor of its own.

Zonite also kills immediately all germs and bacteria on contact. Yet contains no poisons or acids. No other type of liquid antiseptic-germicide is more powerful, yet so safe. Your druggist has Zonite.

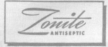

For Every Woman's
Most Serious Deodorant Problem

FREE BOOK
Just Published
Reveals new findings every

This new, frankly-written book reveals up-to-date findings about an intimate problem every woman should understand. Sent in plain envelope. Mail coupon to Dept. 944-P, Zonite Products Corporation, 370 Lexington Avenue, New York 17, N. Y.

Name . . . .

Pity the young wife held back
by false modesty...

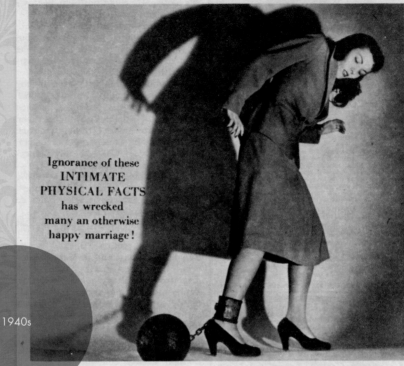

Ignorance of these INTIMATE PHYSICAL FACTS has wrecked many an otherwise happy marriage!

1940s

Often a married woman has no one but herself to blame if her husband starts losing interest—

False modesty may have kept her from consulting her Doctor. Or perhaps she very foolishly has followed *old-fashioned* and *wrong* advice of friends.

If only young wives would realize how important douching two or three times a week often is to intimate feminine cleanliness, health, charm and *marriage happiness.* If only they'd learn about this newer, scientific method of douching with—ZONITE.

No other type liquid antiseptic-germicide tested is SO POWERFUL yet SO HARMLESS
Up-to-date, well-informed women no longer use old-fashioned, weak or dangerous products.

The ZONITE principle is truly a miracle! No other type liquid antisep-tic-germicide for the douche of all those tested is so POWERFUL yet SO SAFE to tissues. Absolutely *non-poisonous, non-burning, non-irritating.* ZONITE positively contains no phenol, no bichloride of mercury, no creosote. You can use ZONITE as directed *as often as needed* without risk of injury.

Zonite Principle Developed By Famous Surgeon and Chemist
ZONITE actually destroys and removes odor-causing waste substances. Helps guard against infection. It's so *powerfully effective* no germs of any kind tested have ever been found that it will not immediately kill on contact. You know it's not always possible to contact all the germs in the tract. BUT YOU CAN BE SURE that ZONITE kills *every reachable* germ and keeps them from multiplying.

Buy a bottle of ZONITE *today!*

Zonite
FOR NEWER
feminine hygiene

FREE! NEW!
For amazing enlightening NEW Booklet containing frank discussion of intimate physical facts, recently published — mail this coupon to Zonite Products, Dept. MO-87, 370 Lexington Ave., New York 17, N. Y.

Name_____

Address_____

City_____ State_____

103

poodle skirts and liked Ike, but routinely shook up bottles of Coca-Cola as an alternative spermicidal douche. And who knew? A good blast of Lysol might terminate an early unwanted pregnancy, as well.

Douching with a stiff dose of Lysol and water was vigorously marketed from the 1920s until the early 1960s, despite the rampant internal scalding and vaginal infections it caused in countless women. Startling as that may sound, the fact is that for decades, none of the douche manufacturers ever bothered to test whether any of their products, with their cartoonishly harsh chemical ingredients, were safe enough for women to keep using every few days.

More recently, the U.S. Department of Health and Human Services, hardly what you'd call a bunch of *Our Bodies, Ourselves* types, has itself recommended against douching because it's a surefire way to kill off all the good-guy bacteria in your vagina. This in turn can easily lead to the bad guys taking over, which can lead to bacterial vaginosis or even pelvic inflammatory disease, which can lead to discomfort, possibly scarring, even infertility . . . and along the way, guess what will happen? *Your vagina will smell really, really bad!* Talk about irony! In fact, even the most innocent-sounding douche of vinegar and water can so imbalance your pH levels, you'll soon be generating enough yeast to open your own bakery. As a result, douching has long since fallen out of favor around the world, except here in the United States, where an estimated 20 to 40 percent of all women still douche regularly.

The Smell Campaign—identifying what could be seen as a problem in the average, healthy vagina, amplifying the average woman's fears about it, and then aggressively marketing products to "fix" it—has been so successful, it's downright scary. In fact, the moment menstrual products came on the market—and to this day—odor has been one of the biggest boogeymen of the so-called feminine hygiene industry . . . the surefire way companies scare you into buying their products. At the same time, it's this very subject, more than any other aspect, that puts its chilly thumb right into the soft, warm belly of the whole femcare advertising paradox. Does anyone honestly think the best way to win over new customers is by openly suggesting they reek to high heaven?

From the very beginning, menstrual advertising has been giving itself the vapors as it struggled to address the Smell Issue. Early copywriters went into flowery overdrive, churning out lavender-scented phrases like "personal daintiness" and "fresh as a daisy," as they struggled to convince women that their product could save them from a lifetime sentence of funk. Euphemisms were tossed about in print ads, with much discreet nudging, meaningful raising of the eyebrows, and diplomatic winking going on.

In those early ads, one could practically hear the creaking anxiety of Modess and Kotex, white-gloved manufacturing doyennes that they were, struggling so very, very hard not to offend. Kotex's earliest tagline was simply "Kotex—protects, deodorizes." (Protects against what? Flying bullets? Malaria?) We especially enjoy the claims of Amolin, a deodorant powder that was quaveringly advertised as being able to get rid of odors "everywhere on the female body." (Like what were you supposed to do . . . gargle with it?)

As with douche ads, the hands-down single best weapon advertisers used—and continue to brandish to this day—was terror; terror of offending, terror of being helplessly awash in stench, terror that admittedly ran a tad toward campiness at times, even luridness, yet was still wildly effective. That's because smell sells.

Consider this 1928 potboiler of an ad for the commercial douche Zonite: "Is a wife to blame if she doesn't know—these intimate physical facts?" We see the wife sobbing as her husband, coat in hand, storms out the door in a huff, nauseated and offended by having to actually breathe air in the same apartment as her vagina. And yet the ad leaves us grateful for the knowledge that for a mere pittance (no more, say, than a packet of tooth powder or the down payment on a new cloche hat), she could win him back!

Okay. So what's the actual story?

Does a healthy vagina in fact emit supercharged smell-o-rama odor rays that can drive men away forever? And does menstrual blood stink to high heaven or doesn't it?

The answer, generally speaking, is "no."

But that being said, the vagina is only human.

While normally possessed of a healthy colony of friendly microorganisms living in odor-free harmony, the vagina still has its off days, especially when presented with

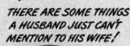
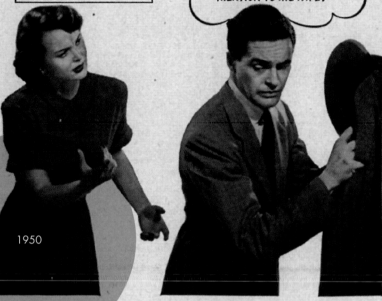

antibiotic use, a sudden change in pH level, noncotton underwear, or unfamiliar semen from a new, condomless partner. Bacterial vaginosis sets in when the not-so-friendly anaerobic bacteria living in one's love canal decide to mutiny and start raising that gigantic family they've always talked about. The smell they ultimately produce is chemically related to the one produced by decomposing bodies, which means some serious funk starts to kicks in; pretty soon, one actually *does* smell like a fish, and definitely not the kind you'd want to order at a restaurant.

We're not doctors, but take it from us: one can pretty much assume that if one suddenly notices any powerful aroma (such as that of low tide or a particularly zesty loaf of bread) emanating from the loins, *this is definitely a warning sign.* It could mean something relatively mild but disheartening, like bacterial vaginosis or a yeast infection. Other than making one feel vaguely like a leper, such low-grade infections are generally no more than an occasionally itchy, clumpy annoyance, and can be dispatched swiftly with topical creams or suppositories.

For the record, it's been proven that bears won't maul you if you have your period.

A horrible new smell could also mean that, silly you, you've forgotten all about that tampon you so blithely inserted days or even weeks ago. While the thought is understandably enough to make anyone blanch, the important thing is to get that mother out, as soon as possible. If for some reason you still can't find it, *calm down;* go see your doctor and remind yourself that this is, in fact, an incredibly common occurrence. If you do end up with an infection, it can most likely be cleared up with antibiotics, and you should end up as good as new.

But vaginal odor can also indicate something more serious, namely pelvic inflammatory disease or even cancer—vaginal, cervical, uterine, bowel—in which case, one

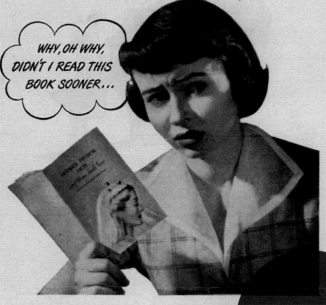
should definitely hightail it to one's gynecologist posthaste, since smelling weird should be the worst of our problems. More rarely, there are unfortunately women who just happen to be born with an imbalance of vaginal flora, which means having a signature aroma.

As for menstrual blood, take it from us: it doesn't smell like anything when it's still inside the body. Even once it's outside, it only takes on a decided bouquet after it's been in contact with air for an extended period of time. We're not whitewashing this one: if you let nature take its course, oxidation will definitely make a used pad pretty damn ripe. Changing regularly, however, is all any pad-wearing female needs to do to settle the question. (And not to spoil your appetite or anything, but one should also keep in mind that the highly touted "wicking" —i.e., absorbing—abilities of today's sanitary napkins will also effectively wick . . . how to put this delicately? . . . bacteria from one's butt.)

But come on, we hear you say . . . of *course* menstrual blood stinks! If I can smell it when I'm changing a tampon, then obviously someone else can smell it, too. And what about camping? What about shark attacks?

In fact, we, too, have college memories of going on camping trips and all of us earnestly grilling each other beforehand: "You don't have your period, do you? You *definitely* don't, right?" We all knew what was bound to happen if one of us was lying . . . some crazed bear or wolverine or coyote would smell the blood and come slavering to get at us! If we were swimming in the ocean, we'd be yanked underwater by a shark and chewed up like a bagel!

As a matter of fact, we weren't just being giddy coeds. For years, the U.S. Parks Department regularly distributed to campers a stern little flyer that was scarier than any Stephen King novel. "Special precautions apply to women!" barked the brochure. "For their protection, women should refrain from wilderness travel during their menstrual periods! Bears and other large carnivores have attacked women in this physiological condition!"

For the record, it's been proven that bears won't maul you if you have your period. In a study using menstruating women and actual bears (which makes us ponder how far we ourselves would go to earn a hundred bucks), eleven females were met with complete apathy by the carnivores, making the experiment seem not unlike speed-dating stories we've heard. For the final touch, another woman wearing a pad not only fed four bears by hand, she then walked within six feet of a group of male bears . . . and they totally ignored her. And to top it all, it was mating season!

When it comes to sharks, it also seems as if the danger is a tad overstated. While sharks have a notoriously keen sense of smell, there's absolutely zero evidence that menstrual blood does anything for them, much less send them ravening in one's general direction. In the book *Diving and Subaquatic Medicine*, the authors speculate that there might be some component in menstrual flow that sharks find off-putting, but what that might be is anyone's guess.

We understandably expect some of you are shaking your heads in disbelief. We just can't get the idea that our periods stink to high heaven out of our heads because that's the way we were raised. But where does this conviction come from, anyway?

The earliest commercial menstrual products were invented in the early twentieth century, and from the beginning, their ads repeatedly reinforced the notion that menstruation was inherently a germ-ridden Mayday, a hygienic disaster that needed at all costs to be wrestled to the ground. To manufacturers, the equation was a delightful no-brainer: if you defined a problem, all you had to do then was add a product and multiply by fear, and hey—presto! The resulting sum equaled sales . . . *lots* of sales.

From the very beginning, tampon makers have boasted that since their product 1943 is worn internally, they've slam-dunked the entire smell issue, unlike the makers of pads. Their missives were often sober and earnest, as befitted such a grave subject (this one from a 1961 Tampax ad): "With a sanitary napkin, the flow collects on the pad where the warmth of the body increases its odor. . . . Many girls prefer to wear tampons . . . since they are worn internally where no air is present: no odor can form." Another ad dutifully reported, "You can avoid menstrual odor entirely . . . when you wear a tampon. Because it is worn internally where no air is present, no odor can form at all."

Yet sanitary pad manufacturers weren't taking this lying down. Outraged, they rose up as one and swiftly began introducing new products specifically formulated to combat odor. Quest, a deodorant powder invented by Kotex in the 1930s, was meant to be liberally

Fresh as a Daisy

Then, here's Part II of our Kotex Kwiz: If Kotex is changed frequently—and great care is taken in bathing—do you know why a deodorant should be used on a sanitary napkin? Science has the answer to that one. It seems that as the menstrual flow leaves the body —it is odorless. But once it reaches the air, odor develops immediately. And, in order to be effective, the deodorant must have direct contact with the flow. That means a *powder* deodorant is needed—sprinkled on the surface of the napkin. Why a powder? Because a powder doesn't interfere with absorption. You may find a cream deodorant well and good for ordinary purposes. But a cream forms a film that slows up absorption. When applied on a sanitary pad, it tends to spread the moisture toward the edges, instead of allowing it to penetrate the bulk of the napkin, as it should.

A positive powder deodorant like Quest (created expressly for napkin use) will banish all body odors completely. And this is important, for odors increase during menstruation. To keep dainty-fresh as a daisy, just remember this simple routine: Every time you change your Kotex (4 or 5 times a day, if possible) . . . sprinkle a little Quest the length of your napkin. You'll be certain to avoid offending. For unscented Quest doesn't cover up one odor with another. It actually destroys odors . . . safely and surely.

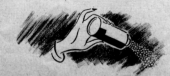

20

Kotex, Kimberly-Clark

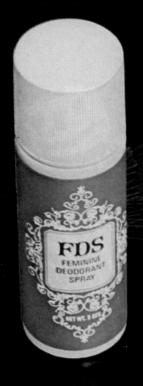

This new product will become as essential to you as your toothbrush.

The name is FDS *
Feminine Hygiene Deodorant Spray.
It is new. A most personal sort
of deodorant. An external
vaginal deodorant.
Unique in all the world.
Essential on special days.
Welcome protection against odor—
every single day.

FDS—for your total freshness.

1966

sprinkled on one's pad prior to use to ensure that ever-crucial "personal daintiness." Educational booklets gave detailed instructions on how to stay clean, how often to change, and how to groom yourself so cunningly that no one could possibly notice the gigantic, lumpy bulge in your crotch.

Tampon makers struck back. In the 1970s, manufacturers started adding perfume to their products. New 'n' improved tampons and pads, both in scented varieties, started flooding the marketplace, practically elbowing one another off the shelves as they fought for their share of the market. Ads touted how wonderful their products smelled! How feminine! How refreshing! A 2004 Procter & Gamble tampon ad depicting a woman in an evening gown lounging elegantly by the water even featured an actual scratch 'n' sniff strip, so you could preview what your lucky vagina could smell like, too!

Like Hatfields and McCoys, tampon and pad manufacturers have been duking it out for decades. After all, when it comes to loyalty, women don't merely attach to brands—when a girl starts with tampons or pads, she's likely to keep using her choice throughout her menstrual life, which adds up to more than thirty-five years. And so the battle rages on.

Today, women are being aggressively sold on "feminine wipes," which bear an uncomfortably close resemblance to the premoistened towelettes mothers everywhere use to wipe the poop off their babies' butts. Flattering comparison, no? Even more ominously, these wipes are actually packaged to resemble those very baby towelettes. One manufacturer even packages individual pads with their own wipes included, so you can wipe yourself clean every time you change a pad, and "feel shower fresh all day." We ourselves are partial to that old standby, toilet paper . . . but where's the profit in that?

What really creeps us out is that more and more women and girls have been complaining of a peculiar, chronic condition that's only recently started to be taken seriously. Called different things, including

Opposite: Alberto Culver Company

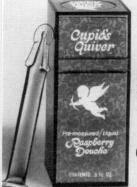

1971

The different douche!

Still using those messy old fashioned medicinal preparations? Get with Cupid's Quiver, the delightfully feminine pre-measured liquid douche that revolutionized douching. Choose from four fabulous fragrances . . . raspberry, champagne, jasmine and orange blossom. Cleanses gently, thoroughly and leaves you refreshingly nice.

At fine drug stores.

Cupid's Quiver™
the gyna-cosmetic

Just curious?
Send $1 for an introductory supply in each of the 4 fragrances: Tawn, Ltd., P.O. Box 448, Dept. L., Bridgeport, Conn. 06602

vulvodynia, vaginal vestibulitis, and "the most painful thing that ever happened to me," it generally consists of inexplicable burning, stabbing discomfort, throbbing and/or itching of the labia or vaginal opening.

Doctors are stumped as to what it is, exactly, or how to treat it. And while it can be brought on by an infection like yeast or herpes, vulvodynia also appears to be triggered by inflammation brought on by soaps, feminine deodorant sprays, perfumes, and commercial femcare products: the very stuff that's supposed to keep us all so dainty.

We're floored that even in these supposedly enlightened times, we're still in thrall to the smell stigma that's held us hostage for so many decades. While the battle over who can scare us more about our stench has been fighting itself out in boardrooms

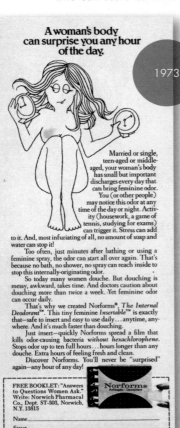

and the stock market, where does that leave us? Apparently, we're left still believing the old arguments that we smell awful, whether we're menstruating or not, and still blithely using products that regularly subject our incredibly sensitive and absorbent labial and vaginal skin to God-knows-what. Companies aren't even required to list the ingredients on their product's packaging and will often just use the catchall word "fragrance."

The perception of odor is one of those subjective things—like having an ear for krunk music, a craving for cilantro, a genuine appreciation for plaid pants. We're not going to tell you what to do with your own body or how we think you should smell, and we sure hope you feel the same way about us. But maybe it's time to reconsider what's being sold so earnestly to all of us, what it might actually be doing to our tender selves, and whether or not we actually want to step in and change the way we shop, the way we keep ourselves clean, the way we perceive ourselves.

Something actually *does* smell kind of funny, doesn't it?

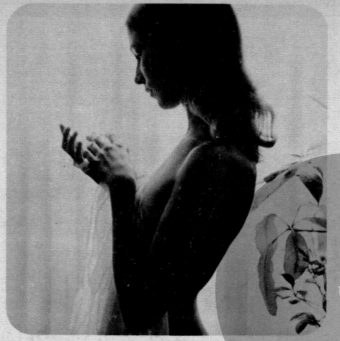

1970s

HAVING A FEMALE BODY DOESN'T MAKE YOU FEMININE.

IT'S THE EXTRA THINGS YOU DO—LIKE FDS.

What is femininity? It's bubble baths. Clean shiny hair. Your favorite perfume. And FDS. The very feminine hygiene deodorant that more girls prefer. Because only FDS has a whole new kind of protection-plus. Two effective deodorants—plus new Time-Release Fragrance Fresheners. Miniature blooms of fragrance that release whenever you're especially active or emotional. Miniature blooms of fragrance that go on working, minute-to-minute, all day long, up to 24 hours. So FDS keeps you feeling fresh and feminine a lot longer.

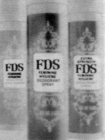

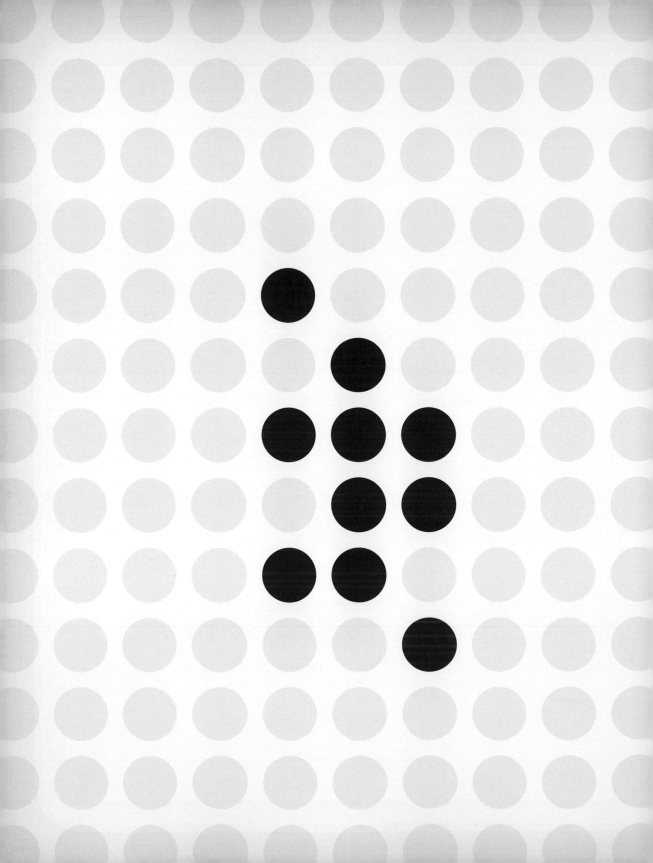

Chapter 10

SO NOW YOU'RE A WOMAN!

Are you there God? It's me, Margaret. Gretchen, my friend, got her period. I'm so jealous, God. I hate myself for being so jealous, but I am. I wish you'd help me just a little. Nancy's sure she's going to get it soon, too. And if I'm last I don't know what I'll do. Oh please God, I just want to be normal.

— *ARE YOU THERE GOD? IT'S ME, MARGARET*

OW MANY HUNDREDS OF THOUSANDS OF GIRLS have waited anxiously to get their chance to read that dog-eared, well-worn copy of Judy Blume's seminal book from 1970, *Are You There God? It's Me, Margaret*, that secretly circulated throughout their school? Passed from friend to friend, talked about in bathrooms, at sleepovers, in notes passed in class, on long phone calls, *Are You There God?* was groundbreaking in that it gave a realistic and identifiable preteen voice to the often confusing experience of growing up.

Through Margaret, girls read about the frustrations of having a body that didn't develop fast enough, the confusion of not fitting in, the fear of being left out and left behind. Blume provided one of the few places girls could get information about menstruation that hit home more profoundly than any lecture in health class or corporate-sponsored film shown in fifth-grade assembly. Her characters talked about what bleeding actually felt like, about crying jags and mood swings, the embarrassment of buying supplies (especially from a boy cashier!), the anxiety of being the last to get one's period.

In 1970, the dialogue about menstruation may have been light-years removed from the tight-lipped exchange that had usually passed for sexual education in previous generations; still, discussing it openly was no walk in the park for either the premenarchal girl or her mother (who was probably toting plenty of her own baggage when it came to repression and embarrassment). Consider the fact that since 1980, Blume's book has been one of the top one hundred books that parents regularly try to have banned from school libraries.

In her 1975 book, *Menstruation & Menopause: The Physiology and Psychology, the Myth and the Reality*, Paula Weideger points out that when a girl hits

One day a little book was put on my bed while I was gone. Next to it were some maxipads and a belt. I assume it was from my mom, but we never talked about it. The book was one of the first editions of Our Bodies, Ourselves, *and I'm pretty sure my mom would have been horrified if she knew what was really in the book.*

—*Beth H.* (46)

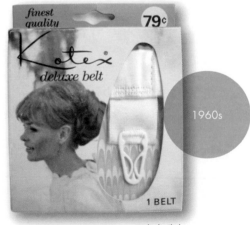

1960s

Kimberly-Clark

puberty, she's pretty much on her own. As her face breaks out, breasts balloon, hair sprouts in weird new places, and emotions carom, she's more often than not sans support as she struggles to understand what's going on and why she has zero control over a body that suddenly appears to be going apeshit. She has no choice but to be swept along—proudly and happily, or kicking and weeping—into adulthood.

Getting one's first period is, of course, one of the most powerful transitions in female life: the flashing light that indicates one is most assuredly leaving the country road of childhood and merging onto the interstate of adulthood. Authors have traditionally pounced on this moment to forcibly remind the lucky young girl of exactly what she's supposed to be feeling, in no uncertain terms. From Mary McGee Williams and Irene Kane's popular *On Becoming a Woman: A Book for Teenage Girls* (1958): "One of the reasons that menstruation sets off an explosion of emotions is that for perhaps the first time in your active, tom-boy life, you must accept the fact that you are a girl. For most girls, this acceptance is an exciting, who-wouldn't-want-to-be kind of thing, something you've looked forward to from the time you saw your mother nursing a baby brother, or dreamed about a kitchen of your own, or imagined yourself a well-loved wife."

McGee Williams and Kane choose not to mention the fact that for other girls, getting one's period is not only confusing and frightening, but often downright depressing as it signals the end of presexual freedom and the joys of childhood itself. Some of us actually enjoyed being active tomboys and were horrified to learn we would now be expected to give up our swashbuckling ways. And in

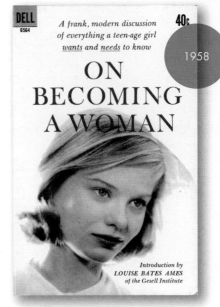

A frank, modern discussion of everything a teen-age girl *wants* and *needs* to know

DELL
6564

40¢

1958

ON BECOMING A WOMAN

Introduction by
LOUISE BATES AMES
of the Gesell Institute

When you have a bat mitzvah you become a woman—at least that's what they tell you in Hebrew school. Which is the same thing they tell you in that fifth-grade film about menstruation: when you get your first period, you're a woman. When I was studying for my bat mitzvah, the two twisted in my head and I started having nightmares that I'd get my first period at my bat mitzvah. I dreamed I was standing up on the bimah, in my short-sleeved white lace gown trimmed with pink satin ribbons, when blood started gushing down my legs. I didn't know what periods were actually like, how much blood you lost, that it didn't happen all at once. In my dreams the blood raged down three steps and into the congregation. Everyone just sat and stared at me. I never told anyone and dreaded my thirteenth birthday—far more afraid I'd bleed in public than screw up my Torah portion.

—*Elissa S.* (43)

fact, first blood isn't even the point of their book, despite its educational-sounding title. While they dutifully spend a grand total of two pages discussing menstruation, the gist of the book consists of chapters like "The Teen-Age Crush," "How to Get—and Keep— Boys Interested," and "It's Not Too Soon to Dream of Marriage."

To say young girls have different reactions to their first period is perhaps the biggest understatement of the century. Yet whether they're over the moon or deeply depressed, scared or elated, all girls are invariably told in no uncertain terms—after all that anticipation and buildup that leads to the first period—to keep their blood to themselves. Save for a best friend or two, no one is ever supposed to know when it's happening, or even if it's happening at all. So what kind of lousy rite of passage is that, anyway?

And yet in other eras and across the world, first bleeding has been treated as something else entirely: as an important, even solemn transition to be celebrated with elaborate rituals and ceremonies. In rural India, a girl was given a ceremonial bath and covered in jewels and special garments before participating in a special ceremony with her family. In Japan, a girl's family still traditionally celebrates her first period by serving red rice and beans. In Sri Lanka, a girl is ritually bathed and dressed in white before being honored at a party, where she receives gifts and money. A Balinese girl is blessed at a temple and is then the guest of honor at a special feast. The Asantes of Ghana also throw a party, replete with singing and dancing, where the girl is given gifts and treated like a queen.

I had been expecting a royal trumpeter to unravel a scroll announcing "its" arrival—turns out there was no regal decree. I simply thought I'd been injured internally somehow and now I was dying slowly. I told my best friend, who confirmed that I was not, in fact, hemorrhaging.

—Lerato S. (37)

These, of course, are the cultures with the fun traditions. Other societies regarded a girl's first period as a more arduous hurdle, the appropriate time for her to prove her physical strength, since she'd obviously need a lot of it as an adult. A Nootka Indian girl would be rowed out to sea and dropped overboard, the expectation being that she'd swim back by herself. Her tribe would wait on shore ready to cheer her return . . . or mount a hasty rescue-and-recover mission.

Some ceremonies lasted for days, even weeks or months. The Mescalero Apaches threw an annual eight-day-long ceremony, the most important of the year, for all girls who started menstruating that year. The first four days were devoted to much public feasting and dancing, while the latter four were set aside for the girls to privately ponder their new status as women. In fact, many cultures believed the time surrounding first menstruation was highly spiritual. Seclusion was considered an invaluable time to meditate, dream, and receive visions, an important part of many puberty rites for both girls and boys.

In Malawi, the Ngoni tribe traditionally secluded each girl for up to three months. Then her face and body would be daubed with white flour, signaling her spiritual and physical split from the community. She sat, naked, in shallow water until the womenfolk determined she could get out and begin her life as a woman. Pygmies in Africa traditionally sent their girls into seclusion to learn about motherhood from an older female relative. Afterward, a celebration was held, often lasting a month or two, so faraway relatives could have time to visit, honor the girl properly, and pay their respects.

According to an old Eastern-European tradition, a mother slaps her daughter across the face when she gets her first period. There are different explanations: to ward off evil spirits, for good luck, to let the girl know the pain of being a woman, or to bring the color back into her cheeks. Whatever the reason, most women who have had it done to them generally remember the moment quite vividly.

As harsh as it may sound, slapping is a walk in the park compared to the rituals other cultures use to mark a girl's entrance into adulthood. In the Tiv tribe in Nigeria, for instance, four lines were traditionally cut in a pubescent girl's abdomen, supposedly to make her more fertile. We don't even want to get into female genital mutilation (FGM), a widely practiced tradition with its roots in North Africa. In FGM, a girl's clitoris and labia are maimed or even removed outright, in an incredibly disturbing ritual practiced on females as young as four all the way up to grown women.

One could argue that even the most extreme ritual exists in the first place because there's something inherently compelling about not only a woman's sexuality, but her monthly blood . . . something powerful, frightening, perhaps even mystical. There have even existed puberty rites for boys that blatantly mimicked menstruation—hands down, the most queasy-making being one called subcision. Subcision, in which the penis was cut along its length so that it bled against the unfortunate boy's lower body, was allegedly a tradition in New Guinea, Australia, the Philippines, and Africa. Blood coming from a sexual organ has clearly been a powerful symbol of adulthood, whether it came about naturally or surgically.

Depending on the culture, the first period has been the cause for celebration or resignation, and has therefore been ritualized, commemorated, or, in our society, basically ignored. While some families manage to muster up a small gift or special dinner, for the most part, American girls get a terse and generic "congratulations, today you are a woman" speech from one or both parents and are pretty much left alone to figure it out for themselves. It's not surprising that the average girl may be totally at sea when it comes to what's going

I was twelve years old. It was summer and I was wearing white Wrangler jeans shorts—the kind we rolled up at the knee. I had a great red-and-white sleeveless gingham top that came just above my waist with ruffles, just like the one Ann-Margret wore in Bye Bye Birdie. I was out on the deck, lying on a chaise with my legs wide open when suddenly, my mother called me to come inside. She pointed out that my beautiful white jeans were stained with deep brownish blood. I was shocked and so embarrassed. We went to the bathroom and when I took off my shorts my mother slapped me, gently, across the face. I freaked out and my mother laughed. She said that it was an old Jewish custom, the slap somehow warded off evil spirits, but I just wanted to cry. She explained that her mother slapped her, too. It was something every mother did when her daughter got her first period. Years later, I was glad that I had a son. That would have been a tough custom to carry on.

—Stephanie F. (53)

on with her changing body, what to expect, what's normal, and how she should feel about it all in the first place.

So what's going on with that first period, anyway?

The technical term for the onset of menstruation is "menarche," which stems from the Greek words *mene* (meaning "moon") and *arche* ("beginning"). Ancient civilizations took note of how the monthly cycles of the moon seemed to mirror women's monthly bleeding; and today, we ourselves find basing such a word on moon imagery quite poetic, even if the final result sounds disturbingly like "malarkey."

Puberty, the physical transformation from girl to adult, takes about four years altogether. It's made up of three consecutive stages, each one often the source of great pride, distress, confusion, or all three: breast budding, growth of pubic hair, and, finally, menarche. Back in 1830, the average age for a girl's first blood was seventeen. Today, however, the average age is between 12.8 and 13.2 years, although anywhere between nine and seventeen is considered normal.

What exactly triggers menarche is still hotly debated. Some think it's brought on by a certain accumulation of fat; others point to skeletal growth. Whatever the precise cause, it's

1940

What is menstruation?

MENSTRUATION is the normal periodic flow of blood from the uterus. It occurs periodically—at regular intervals. That is why menstruation is often called a "period."

At what age does menstruation begin?

Most American girls begin to menstruate between the ages of 11 and 16. Some may begin a little earlier; some may begin a little later. A number of things may affect the exact age when menstruation begins. Among them are heredity, general health, environment, climate, etc.

It is generally believed that girls in tropical countries, for example, begin to menstruate earlier than girls in cold climates.

4

The Periodic Cycle, Modess, Johnson & Johnson

widely believed that improved nutrition and environmental conditions over the years are what gradually brought the age of menarche down to where it is today.

Ironically, early menarche puts women at a higher risk for cancer, particularly breast cancer, since it exposes the girl to extra estrogen in her lifetime. And creepily enough, there are now ominous signs that the earliest sign of puberty, breast budding, is occurring at younger and younger ages, perhaps due to the so-called obesity epidemic, hormones in our diet, the presence of environmental pollutants, or any combination of the three. Whether or not this affects the age of menarche or a girl's overall health is still completely unknown.

Early pregnancy fears aside, menarche isn't necessarily a sign of immediate fertility; in fact, it can take a couple of years not only for a regular cycle to establish itself but also for ovulation to rev up. That being said, menarche has been widely used in many if not most cultures as the sign that a girl is ready to hit the marriage market, and that motherhood, her basic reason for even existing in the first place, is pretty much nigh at hand.

From that day on, my mother was watching over me like a hawk, and often, whenever there was talk about a boy, or she would see me with a boy, she would say something like "don't get pregnant" or "you know that you can get pregnant now."

—Cassandra P. (51)

As a result, menarche has also routinely kicked off the time of training the hapless girl so she could handle the responsibilities that would soon be piled upon her slim shoulders. Whether it was a Native American girl drafted into puberty rites, a frontier adolescent learning how to bake bread, or a debutante-to-be being strapped into her first corset, menarche has traditionally marked the definitive end of girlhood, and the start of some heavy expectations.

Twenty-first-century Americans tend to gloss over the event, skittering around any personally meaningful acknowledgment of the physical and emotional changes going on and instead handing off the hapless girl into the waiting arms of the commercial femcare industry. That's the downer part. The positive part is that there's vastly more information available to the confused adolescent than ever before, and it's easily accessible online and in girls' magazines, too: not only the basic anatomical facts, but even practical tips on how to insert a tampon for the first time and deal with cramps.

Of course, much if not all of that information is provided by the femcare manufacturers, and as saintly and altruistic as some of them may be as individuals, they in fact all share a not-so-secret common agenda, which is to sell their stash. After all, we gals tend to be brand loyalists, especially when it comes to our tampon and pad choices. If a company can successfully woo a preteen, it also gains a potential lifelong customer. As a result, young girls barely beyond Barbie are routinely bombarded with femcare ads, articles, and advice in teen magazines and on the Internet.

So is this really so awful? We sure as hell don't know. All we do know is that there's often a highly convoluted dance in teen magazines, in both their articles and advertisements, between good information and constructive tips, and prudish, even repressive advice. Sexy outfits modeled by apparent jailbait will nestle up against articles warning girls "not to go too far."

The same thing holds true for teen magazines and their take on menstruation. A perfectly sensible letter about whether it's possible to get pregnant during one's period will be answered in reasonable detail, but it will then be followed by a short story detailing the lurid downfall of a girl who foolishly "let" her boyfriend "go all the way." This will then be followed by a bouncy, full-page ad extolling the undetectability of a new pad or the flowery scent of a new tampon.

Much of the weird tension between actual information and prudishness and shame in teen magazines and femcare Web sites arises from the complex history of menstrual education. Throughout most of history, it was a mother's job to teach her daughters about menstruation . . . or at least, that was the way it was supposed to work *in theory*. In fact, many if not most mothers shied away from that delicate task and as a result, even in recent years, countless girls have experienced their first period with no real understanding of what was going on and were understandably scared to death to discover reddish-brown sludge in their knickers.

For centuries, menstrual ignorance ran rampant, unchecked by science, facts, or even shared information. And so it was a truly enlightened move back in the nineteenth

Somewhere out there is an entire store full of chocolate.

Road trip!

Have a happy period.

2008

That time of the month? Let's raise the bar on

high maintenance.

Have a happy period.

always.

E-cards, Procter & Gamble Company

century, when the first intrepid educators squared their jaws and resolutely set about informing girls about menstruation and fertility. Of course, getting down to the actual facts took a certain amount of revving up:

> And now, my dear reader, if you never knew before, you
> must by this time understand what is meant by being "born."
> You now know that the dear little babies that come to our homes
> are not brought there by angels, or by storks, or by doctors.
> They are not found in the woods, or in hollow stumps,
> or in birds' nests, or in hay-mows.
> — *CONFIDENTIAL TALKS WITH YOUNG WOMEN* (1898)

Such books were meant as handy tools to give tongue-tied mothers an easy way to start those gentle, womanly conversations, with the facts conveniently at their soft, white fingertips. As a result, early educators didn't start off their books with graphic descriptions of menstruation or reproduction; no sir, they began where any gentleman would, which is with the fertilization of plants. The theory was that by discussing acorns, apple trees, and marigolds and then nonchalantly working their way up through the animal kingdom, they could maybe slip human intercourse in there along the way without anyone being unduly alarmed.

Back then, the not-so-hidden agenda woven throughout nearly all of these early so-called educational books was basically how menstruation tied in with a girl's expected role as future wife and mother. Menstruation, marriage, motherhood: throughout most of history, these were the three Ms that pretty much summed up the lucky girl's future.

I was thirteen, in eighth grade. I knew about it ahead of time, but it was so conceptual to me that when it finally came, I thought I was bleeding to death. I sat down in the washroom (I was at home with my parents and siblings) and saw that I was gushing blood. I didn't immediately think "menstruation" but rather, "I'm dying!" So I screamed out from the washroom to my parents downstairs, "Call an ambulance—I'm bleeding!" and I could hear peals of laughter in response, which further contributed to my confusion and growing panic.

—Kate R. (47)

And lest any girl dare to actually dream of becoming something other than wife and mother, McGee Williams and Kane, in *On Becoming a Woman*, were there to gently, kindly bitch-slap her back into reality, citing her monthly blood: "What do the changes indicate? You're a girl and you are getting ready for the special role of childbearing. Like every other woman in the world, this is what your body was planned for. You may think you were intended to be a Hollywood star, or a scientist, or a great writer. But your body ignores all this. . . . In childbirth, a woman . . . is creative in a very real sense because she helps create and nourish human beings. . . . When you know the happiness of childbirth—you will be acting the role you were created for."

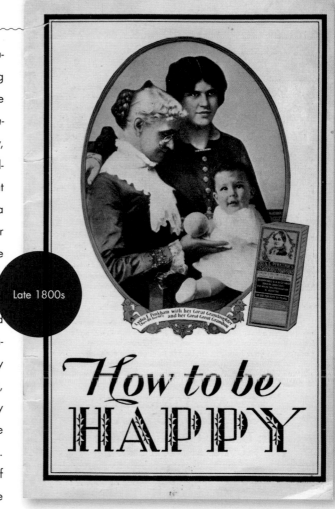

Late 1800s

Lydia E. Pinkham Medicine Company

Despite these baby steps in education, there was never a word in any of these early publications about *what to actually do with all that menstrual flow!* Chapters on hygiene generally went on and on about perspiration (bad), the right way to draw a bath (good, as long as the water was not too hot and certainly never too cold), as well as the pros and cons of whether or not it was okay to wash one's hair (mixed to bad). But before commercial products were commonly available, there was nary a word written on rag wrapping, packing, pinning, or washing, leaving girls at a relative loss as to what to do.

All this changed when the burgeoning femcare industry realized that in order to survive, it had better get into the menstrual education business, as well, and posthaste. It was only a matter of time until manufacturers realized that they could in fact toss their marketing net even wider—and take aim at not just the menstruators, but the prepubertal set. What better way to build brand loyalty than by helping mothers help their daughters? How cozy was that?

Manufacturers started cranking out booklets like "How Shall I Tell My Daughter?" and "Marjorie May's Twelfth Birthday," designed to help mothers talk to their daughters by providing information about menstruation and puberty in one easy-to-read place. The booklets oozed not only empathetic support for the brave mother, but also plenty of hard-sell information about their products. In fact, these booklets were little more than advertising wrapped in high-minded education: an early-twentieth-century version of the infomercial.

My mother showed me these pamphlets, "Growing Up and Liking It" and "What Every Girl Should Know." They each had these cutaway side views of the female reproductive system. I thought getting your period meant having to cut off one leg. Then she took me to a Disney film from Girl Scout group that showed what menstruation was. None of it made any sense.

—Elizabeth O. (52)

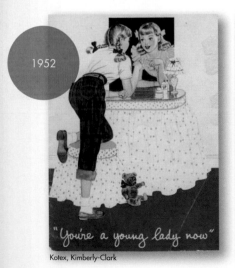

1952

"*You're a young lady now*"

Kotex, Kimberly-Clark

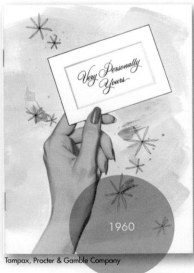

1960

Tampax, Procter & Gamble Company

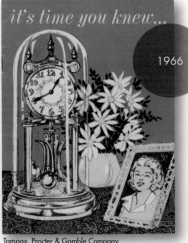

it's time you knew...

1966

Tampax, Procter & Gamble Company

In the 1920s, femcare companies dished out free samples and booklets like candy corn on Halloween. The woman-to-woman faux educational tone seeped into their print ads, as well:

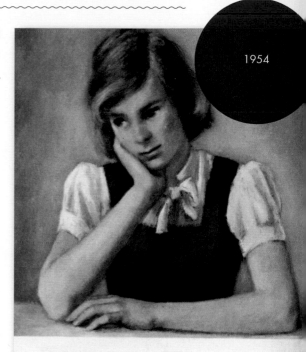

1954

H ow Shall I Tell My Daughter?

Modess, Johnson & Johnson

Blonde: *"Whenever I think over the handicaps nature handed to women, I just boil."*

Brunette: *"I wouldn't talk that way, Fran, especially not around a young daughter."*

Blonde: *"That's just what riles me. Here Grace is just twelve, and has to go through this miserable uncomfortable time—rubbing . . . chafing . . ."*

Brunette: *"Why Fran, dear, why don't you get that child a box of the new Kotex. It's as soft as down."*

—KOTEX AD (1926)

But why go through a motherly middleman? Femcare companies quickly figured out it made more sense to market directly to the girls themselves. In one swift move, menstrual education was effectively yanked from the hands of mothers and taken over by commercial manufacturers.

Schools became the new venue for educating new generations of shoppers, with menstruation now comfortably marketed as an issue of hygiene, not fertility. Femcare manufacturers began producing not only promotional booklets, but short films, as well. While the hairstyles, music, and fashion have changed over time, these films have followed the same structure for decades: after a clinical description of the menstrual cycle and female reproductive anatomy, including information on hygiene, hormones, and physical changes during puberty, every film ends with a "how-to" that shamelessly plugs the sponsor's product. Even Walt Disney produced an animated film for Kotex in the 1940s, in which adolescents who bore an eerie resemblance to Cinderella and Snow White pondered the mysteries of growing up.

A girl and her parents had no choice over which educational film she'd be shown in fifth-grade assembly; the femcare companies, after all, dealt directly with the schools themselves. And the competition occasionally grew a tad testy, especially when it came to the question of which was the best product for young girls: pads or tampons?

The pro-tampon arguments flew like right hooks in a bare-knuckled prizefight:

> *There are two odor problems you can have during your period. One is body odor—for you perspire more profusely during your period. That is why daily baths are so important and deodorants should be used. The other problem is menstrual odor—which may form when pads are worn. You can avoid menstrual odor entirely, however, when you wear a tampon.*
>
> —"ACCENT ON YOU," TAMPAX BOOKLET (1966)

And:

> *Bulky, soiled pads should never be flushed down the toilet, as this often clogs the plumbing. It is best to wrap them in paper and dispose of them discreetly. On visits, this isn't always convenient. That's one reason many girls turn to tampons which, because of their small size, are easily flushed away.*
>
> —"ACCENT ON YOU," TAMPAX BOOKLET (1966)

The pad makers countered with the knockout punch, the ultimate roundhouse blow:

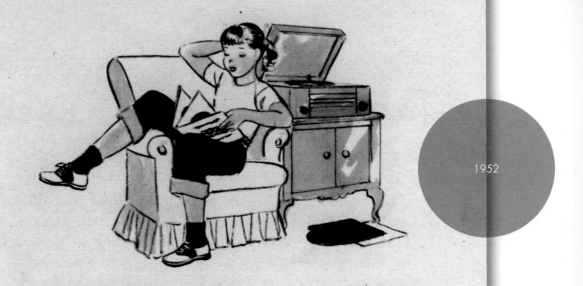

How will you feel?

Pay no attention to a little ache or two but be sure to tell your mother about any real discomfort.

If you should happen to feel a bit low, maybe a nap would cheer you up. Or take your mind off your middle by going to the movies . . . reading an interesting book . . . playing your favorite records . . . joining the other girls at whatever they are doing.

Since you can expect these few days every month, you can learn to live with them easily. They needn't upset you. After all, menstruation is so right and normal. Once you understand it and how little bother it need be, paying attention to it makes about as much sense as worrying over your breathing.

You're a Young Lady Now, Kotex, Kimberly-Clark

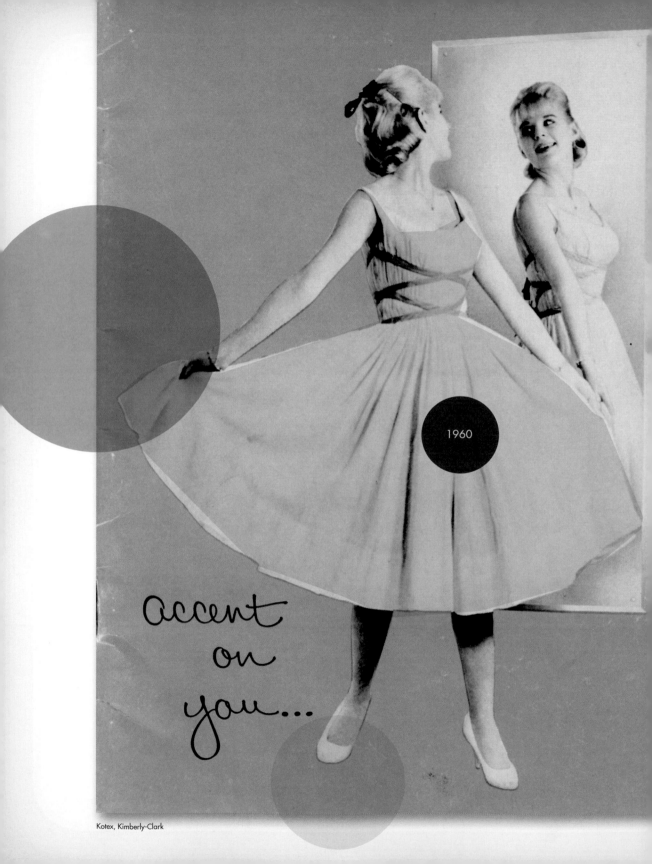

1960

Accent on you...

Well, frankly, most authorities say young girls shouldn't use tampons without first consulting their doctors. The reason is this. In most girls, there's usually a membrane called the hymen, which partly closes the entrance to the vagina—from which comes the menstrual flow. Therefore, Kotex sanitary napkins are much more comfortable, and better suited to a young girl's needs, than tampons of any type.

—"AS ONE GIRL TO ANOTHER," KOTEX BOOKLET (1943)

It turned out that many people, including priests in the Catholic Church, honestly believed that not only were tampons potentially sexually arousing, far more seriously, when a girl inserted one for the first time, she would tear her hymen and lose her virginity. It's astounding how many girls still believe this particular myth; as recently as 1990, Tampax ran an ad with the headline, "Are You Sure I'll Still Be a Virgin?" In fact, the hymen is a stretchy little devil that doesn't even totally cover the vagina (think about it: how could the blood get out otherwise?). And even in the incredibly rare instance of a girl actually tearing her hymen by inserting a tampon, what's the big deal? After all, the only way anyone loses her virginity is through sexual intercourse, remember?

It was just after my twelfth birthday and I felt a gross, wet sensation in my underwear and pain in my lower back. I knew what was going on. I got a pad out of the closet by the bathroom and stuck it in. I called my mom at work. She got me a plant.

—Sophie M. (21)

We appreciate commercially available femcare, we truly do; yet we are disturbed that by allowing manufacturers and their advertisers to be the ones to educate our pubescent daughters, nieces, and granddaughters about this crucial moment in their lives, we are instead letting them use shame and embarrassment freely, for the sole purpose of creating lifelong customers. With them, we have become complicit in treating menstruation as a monthly biological event we buy supplies for, and nothing more.

What does it say about our society that all social, spiritual, and cultural significance has been, well, bled out of menarche?

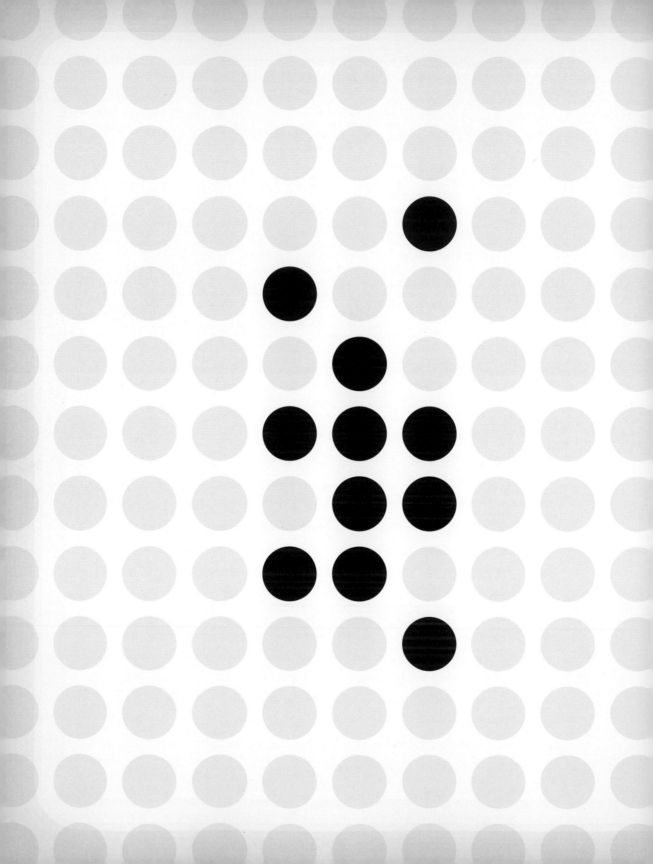

Chapter 11

BACK TO BASICS

MENSTRUATION IS A FUNNY PROCESS IN THAT it's perhaps the only regular bodily event that is, more often than not, greeted with powerful emotion. At this very moment around the world, you can bet that countless females (and not a few of their significant others) are praying feverishly for the appearance of that telltale blood, or else dreading it with a heavy heart. In comparison, one doesn't generally see people weeping with either relief or despair over, say, the sloughing of dead skin cells off their elbow, the growth of a new toenail, a bowel movement, or a good sneeze. Yet getting her period is something that can easily make a grown woman burst into racking sobs . . . or kick up her heels and order a fresh round of drinks for the house.

"*I'm late!*"

Is there a woman alive who doesn't understand that particular code, perhaps one of the most resonant two-word phrases in our universal dictionary?

For heterosexually active females of childbearing age, menstruation has always served one immensely practical purpose: it's the universal indicator that one is not pregnant . . . not *yet*, at any rate. Unlike the light spotting that pregnant women occasionally experience, a genuine three-to-five-day flow is about as clear a signal as you can get from your body that conception is still, at the very least, another cycle away.

Funnily enough, using one's flow to determine whether or not one is pregnant is also where most women's understanding of the whole process begins—and ends. The problem is not only that this is a severely limited definition of a decidedly complex and downright mysterious event, it isn't even that accurate, either. The fact is, a woman can and often does menstruate without ovulating, and vice versa. Up to 80 percent of the menstrual cycles that occur during the first two years of a girl's reproductive life happen without ovulation taking place. Similarly, older women in the later stages of perimenopause often have periods without ovulating, as well. On the flip side, it's incredibly common for an amenorrheic woman, that is, someone who hasn't had her period in months, to get pregnant, because despite her lack of menstrual flow, she was actually ovulating all along.

Even today, there's astoundingly bad education about fertility, reproduction, and basic human physiology, resulting in widespread misinformation, confusion, and fear— even among people who should know better. We are routinely moved and appalled by the basic details so many teenage girls and young women don't seem to know: that urine and menstrual flow emerge from two totally different openings, the urethra and the vagina, for example, or that having unprotected sex the week after one's period is akin to begging to get knocked up.

To make matters worse, ignorance is clearly not just an issue for the very young. Overwhelmingly, women in their twenties and even seasoned old broads have many of the same questions that their prepubertal sisters have about this most basic of female functions. Many of these questions revolve around a shared yet unspoken fear, a prickling, secret suspicion that one is, in fact, a biological anomaly, some kind of medical freak: Is something wrong with me? Is this normal? Why is my cycle so irregular? Why are my cramps so painful/nonexistent, my flow so heavy/light, my mood so awful/elated? Am I having a miscarriage? Is something wrong with me?

To be fair, what we still don't know about menstruation could fill a small library. The big think tanks, universities, and research labs don't traditionally spend any time, thought, or money on the hows and whys of normal, nonpathological menstruation. As a result, there's a limit to how much we know definitively.

What's more, menstruation is in fact a fairly unusual event in the natural world. As we mentioned earlier, other than humans, only some other primates and, weirdly enough, a few lucky bats and shrews get to menstruate at all. Contrary to popular belief, female dogs and cats don't menstruate. Sure, some may bleed a little when in heat—which is why one occasionally catches the odd sight of that scary Rottweiler sporting a doggie menstrual pad—but they don't undergo any of the cyclical hormonal and physiological changes that constitute a real period. Of the select group of menstruating mammals, humans also overwhelmingly bleed the most, far more than even the great apes.

As one probably remembers all too well from that film we were shown in the fifth grade, during the menstrual cycle, a human female produces one or more mature eggs, as her body gets locked and loaded in preparation for pregnancy. This is, however, a pretty singular event in the animal kingdom. There are other kinds of female adaptations when it comes to reproduction, the most common being "seasonal ovulation."

In seasonal ovulation, female animals periodically enter a condition known as "estrus" or, if you're feeling folksy, "being in heat." For these animals, their menstrual cycle actually starts before estrus. The uterine lining starts growing, ovulation occurs, and estrus finally kicks in. Estrus is the only time such a female will be even remotely interested in sex, and she will emphatically give any male the bum's rush if he attempts to pitch woo at another time.

In some animals, an actual physical barrier prevents sex from occurring at any time outside of estrus, acting like a kind of Darwinian chastity belt. For instance, the vagina of a female guinea pig is usually protected by an impenetrable membrane, but exposure to estrogen and progesterone during ovulation makes it magically open up, not unlike Aladdin's cave, to the lucky male guinea pig. This is not only an effective means of maximizing the investment of sex, but is also a terrific conversation starter at your next cocktail party. Similarly, unless a female rat is in heat, her ovaries don't secrete any sex hormones, either. And without them, she can't assume the saucy position known as "lordosis," in which she arches her back and flips her tail aside invitingly, allowing the right male access to her rodent-y charms.

Other animals (most familiarly, cats and rabbits, but also camels, ferrets, the short-tailed tree shrew, and minks . . . who knew?) are what's called reflex ovulators. For them, ovulation is actually triggered by the physical stimulation of intercourse, which makes this perhaps the most efficient way for mammals to reproduce. It's only female primates, including humans, who can literally have sex anytime they want—without ovulation having just occurred beforehand, and without triggering ovulation in the process, either.

In a small study of women in New York City, 61 percent said they had had a period when they weren't expecting it . . . and we bet the others were lying.

There is, however, an interesting fertility notion floating about that an orgasm can actually cause a woman to ovulate right there on the spot, which would effectively make her a reflex ovulator. Could this possibly be true? In her 1999 book, *Woman: An Intimate Geography*, Natalie Angier ruminates on the observation that a woman is, in fact, somewhat likelier to become knocked up from sex with an excitingly adulterous lover, rather than with a lawful, presumably boring, husband.

While perhaps the underlying fantasy is that a man's sexual prowess can be so overwhelming that it can cause even eggs to swoon right then and there, there simply hasn't been enough research done in this area to prove or disprove this intriguing theory. As far as we know, the process that leads to menstruation is a complex cycle of hormones regularly released over a period of time, month after month, as well as their interplay with organs—not just the obvious reproductive ones, but others throughout the body.

In most animals, if sex doesn't result in conception, the uterine lining is simply reabsorbed. In humans, however, it's expelled down through the vagina and out the body—on average, every twenty-eight days. This, however, is a rough average. What's considered "normal" can and will range anywhere from twenty days to forty-five, even in one's own lifetime.

In a small study of women in New York City, 61 percent said they had had a period when they weren't expecting it . . . and we bet the others were lying. Unless you're on the Pill and are therefore experiencing that phony-baloney, regular-as-clockwork pseudo-period, perfect menstrual regularity is not unlike sightings of the Loch Ness monster or Bigfoot, rumored to exist but rarely experienced in person. Hitting one's mark within three to four days is the best most women get—and that usually only happens in one's twenties and thirties. Even twenty-seven-year-old Joan Benoit Samuelson, winner of the first women's marathon in the 1984 Olympics, ran with a just-in-case tampon pinned to the inside of her shorts. If you're in your teens or forties, your cycle will most likely occur in wildly irregular nonpatterns, flummoxing one and all. And for some reason, flight attendants seem to have it the worst—they not only have the heaviest flow, but the greatest irregularity.

At the same time, while the length of a cycle may vary wildly from month to month over the course of one's life, and from woman to woman, the actual sequence of events that take place within the cycle is amazingly constant.

Do you remember that strange diagram of the female reproductive organs from those movies they showed girls in junior high, the one that so eerily resembled a moose's head? To us, the uterus and ovaries, projected up there on that giant screen, seemed at least as big as a toaster oven. It's downright disconcerting for us to realize that, in fact, the uterus is only about three inches long, and weighs a mere two ounces. Held loosely in place by ligaments, it dangles jauntily in one's pelvis like a sailor in his hammock, tipping and shifting depending on whether one is standing, sitting, lying down, or doing the plow position in yoga class.

The two ovaries are small, vaguely resemble lumpy grapes, and are, at least when you're young, chock-full of egg cells. And while the shelf life on human eggs is distinctly better than that of a carton of chicken eggs you get at the supermarket, it's still incredibly limited and inflexible: pretty much fifty years for all women, throughout time, despite any and all advances in diet, medical care, and technology. From one's mid-thirties onward, one's egg cells start to degenerate faster than potato salad on a hot day. By fifty, no matter who you are and how much of a health nut you've been your whole life, those egg cells are pretty much outta there, long gone, a distant memory. Compare this to when a girl is born—she starts off with about one to two million egg cells. Yet by the time she hits menarche, it's already down to 300,000.

The ovaries are on either side of the uterus and, like two tough customers from an old gangster movie, are literally covered with scars—one for each time an egg follicle has ruptured, releasing a mature egg during ovulation. The ovaries also produce hormones, the most important being estrogen and progesterone.

The first day of your flow is also, conveniently enough, considered day one of your menstrual cycle. This is when the hypothalamus, that almond-size gland way up in your brain, sends out a hormonal message to its neighboring gland, the pituitary, which then sends out a chemical message of its own, the follicle stimulating hormone (FSH), down to the ovaries. Like the final recipient in a game of Telephone, about twenty follicles and their eggs in one ovary (and the ovaries take turns ovulating, from month to month) thus get the cue to start ripening.

On day ten, only one follicle of the original twenty is allowed to continue developing; if two do so and pregnancy occurs, fraternal twins could be the result. As this follicle grows bigger, its egg matures. In the meantime, the other nineteen follicles and their egg cells dry up and die (which helps explain what happens to at least some of those eggs you were born with). By now, the feathery, hairy tissue tips of the fallopian tubes have begun eagerly caressing the ovary in anticipation of the big O, ovulation itself.

Sure enough, on day thirteen or thereabouts, the pituitary gland up in the brain squirts out another chemical message, the luteinizing hormone, which now tells the fully ripened follicle it's time to ovulate. Since the ovary doesn't have any openings, the follicle splits open—which can cause *mittelschmerz*, the decidedly unpleasant twinge, cramping, or occasional spotting many women experience midcycle—and the egg is pushed out into the waiting tips of one of the fallopian tubes. Over the next few hours, it will travel through that tube, hooking up with any sperm that happens to be hanging around, even from sex that occurred several days earlier. That's because while an egg is alive for only about twenty-four hours after ovulation, sperm can last a lot longer—anywhere from three to five days, sometimes even more. As a result, a woman is fertile for the time surrounding ovulation for a total of about a week to ten days in the middle of her cycle.

With the egg safely on its way, what's left of the ruptured, left-behind follicle secretes the hormones progesterone and estrogen. These in turn signal the lining of the uterus to grow.

The lining of the uterus (aka the endometrium) is made up of three layers of mucous membrane. Mucus, for your information, is not just the gooey stuff you blow out of your nose on occasion, but is in fact an important secretion made up of a protein, salts, and water. The top two layers are built on top of the bottom layer, which acts as a base. They're supplied with blood through three arteries; if a woman becomes pregnant, the egg will attach to the uterine wall, and these arteries will continue to stock the placenta with blood.

But if the usual state of affairs occurs and conception doesn't take place, the egg either dissolves or gets absorbed into the body. Hormone production abruptly ends, and progesterone and estrogen levels plummet. As a result, the day before flow is due to start, those three arteries cut off blood flow to the uterus, in effect killing off those top two layers of endometrial tissue. Then suddenly, *wham*, they briefly open up again like a fire hydrant, allowing blood to rush in under the dead tissue, basically forcing it to explode.

And where does it all go? You guessed it—motored by gravity and cramps, it all goes down through your cervix and out of your vagina, that's where! Cramps are basically uterine contractions, the kind that can ultimately propel squirming babies out into the waiting world.

This, then, is menstrual flow—the mysterious stuff people have been making such an unholy racket over all these centuries. All told, it's only about two to three ounces, or four to six tablespoons' worth, of blood, mucus, and uterine tissue. That's all menstrual flow is. Made up of familiar ingredients any woman has lying around her body, it's not inherently poisonous, dangerous, or teeming with weird diseases. The blood is identical to the same old blood that comes out of your finger when you accidentally stab it with a bagel knife, with one exception—since it has relatively few platelets, menstrual blood doesn't clot. Those impressive clumps occasionally found in one's flow aren't actually congealed blood, but bits of uterine tissue from those top two endometrial layers.

So if you do the math from day one (the first day of your period), you'll notice that ovulation takes place about two weeks later. But since sperm can hang around in your fallopian tubes for several days waiting for some action, this means that the *two weeks or so after your period ends* is an especially fertile time. Having sex during your flow doesn't mean you won't get pregnant, either. For one thing, it might not actually be a period, but the occasionally heavy spotting many women get at ovulation, i.e., their most fertile time. What's more, it's possible for women with extremely short or, weirdly enough, very long cycles to be ovulating much closer to the time of actual bleeding. If you really don't want to get pregnant, just make sure to use protection every time you have sex.

This elaborate Kabuki dance of glands, hormones, eggs, and follicles is, of course, totally missing when one is on the Pill. During the three weeks one is ingesting the active estrogen or estrogen/progestin-containing pills of one's packet, the hapless body is chemically hoodwinked into thinking that it's pregnant. Mission seemingly accomplished, it then feels no need for its usual hormonal Morse code relay from brain to uterus, that crazy monthly Battle of the Eggs, ovulation itself, the fallopian wide receiver catching the egg and transmitting it to the uterus. Being on the Pill essentially

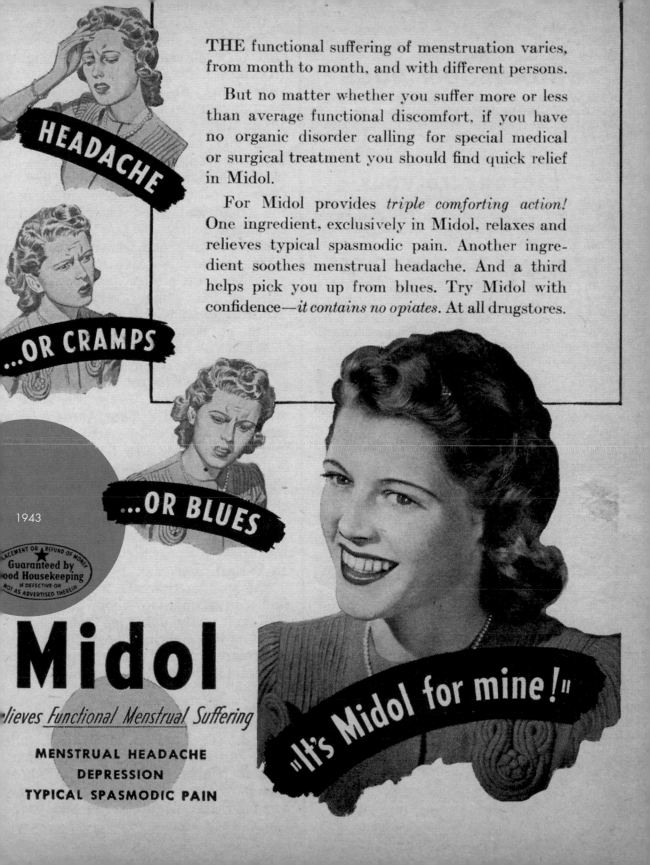

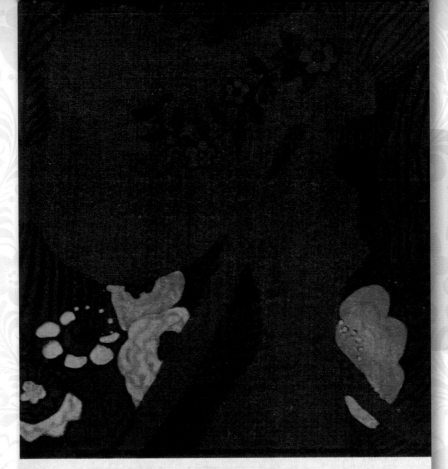

Come discover
Kotique feminine pain relievers

The "liberation" every woman wants

1971

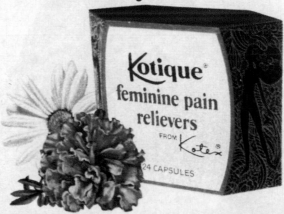

suppresses the ovaries' function, which may explain why it also significantly decreases the risk of ovarian cancer. Furthermore, while there is a mild building up of the endometrium during this time brought on by the low levels of synthetic hormones, it's nothing like the usual heavy feeding of the dense, blood-gorged nest waiting for implantation. All of this explains why one's period—the flow, the cramping, the symptoms—is invariably so much milder when one is on the Pill than not: because it isn't really a period at all.

And speaking of menstrual symptoms . . . what's up with that, anyway? Why do those of us not on the Pill have to put up with all the bloating, backache, constipation? Why do women with normally perfect skin suddenly sprout giant zits, and why do ladies with impeccable manners overnight develop uncontrollable flatulence? What's with the headaches, the cramps? In fact, menstruation is unique in that it's pretty much the only bodily process in which mild to rather severe discomfort is considered part of normal functioning.

To be fair, menstruation is also routinely linked to mood swings, anger, euphoria, horniness, energy, and creativity. Few, however, choose to dwell on any positive aspects. So how much of our monthly ordeal is made worse by our own expectations? How much of it is real? And if it is real, why isn't it the same for all women? And what causes it, anyway?

It's important to remember that menstruation isn't simply a matter of a little blood four days a month, end of story. In fact, virtually every part of one's body is affected during every stage of a normal menstrual cycle, i.e., 365 days a year: pulse rate, blood pressure, body temperature, even the frequency of urination. That being said, there are definitely menstrual symptoms that are common to many if not most women: weight gain, food cravings, cramps, bloating. Unfortunately, there are very few hard answers as to exactly what causes many of these symptoms. All we seem to know is that they most likely arise somehow from normal hormonal fluctuations and cyclical changes in our brain chemistry.

For example, many women report they have an especially intense craving for carbohydrates, sugar, and desserts in the later part of their cycles, during the premenstrual time. Exactly why this is hasn't yet been proven (although does anyone really need a reason to crave a brownie?). Some theorize that the body responds more strongly to insulin right before one's period due to high hormone levels, which results in lowered blood sugar. Still, no one knows for certain.

The week before a period is also when many women get sore, tender breasts. This may be because the same hormones—progesterone and estrogen—busily pumping out of that ruptured follicle of yours aren't just stimulating your uterus and making its lining grow; they're also stimulating your poor, hapless breasts, leaving them achey and swollen.

Others say that breast pain is caused by bloating. Bloating is an incredibly common and vaguely unpleasant symptom in which one's stomach, hands, breasts, and feet blow up to often comical proportions, making one feel not unlike a balloon in the Macy's Thanksgiving Day Parade. Bloating occurs when fluids that normally flow merrily along with one's blood get trapped in and around tissue cells. The pressure within a cell is controlled by electrolytes like sodium; the more sodium in one's body, the more fluid from one's blood makes its way into the cells and is trapped there, like teeny-weeny balloons filled with too much water. And in fact, the higher levels of estrogen and progesterone in the preperiod stage may cause the body to retain sodium—which would definitely lead to that unattractive scenario.

Another theory about bloating is that in many women, the normal premenstrual surge of estrogen triggers the production of *another* hormone, aldosterone. Among other things, aldosterone is known to cause the kidneys to retain fluids. Whatever the reason, bloating means that many premenstrual women can pack on up to six pounds of water gain each month—about the same as dragging around a medium-size dumbbell or a smallish cat. You can help things out by avoiding sugar, starch, salt, booze, and, ironically enough, by drinking more water. Potassium also seems to help get rid of water retention, so try grabbing a banana or some raisins instead of that pecan pie you may well be eyeing by now. Exercise and calcium supplements also seem to help ease the bloat factor for many.

We're sad to report that those fluctuating hormones also appear to wreak havoc on one's gastrointestinal tract, causing everything from constipation and uncomfortable gas to diarrhea. Again, the exact how and why of all this is still not clear. It may have something to do with the hormones that cause the uterus to contract; it's possible that they make the smooth muscle in the intestines contract, as well.

If you're unfortunate enough to be one of the eighteen million women who suffer from migraines, there's a good chance that you also suffer from menstrual migraines, migraines that come during your period. Menstrual migraines are especially severe and don't respond to medication. They're mostly caused by the sudden drop in estrogen right before the start of flow. Many sufferers report that their attacks disappeared during pregnancy. The Pill also seems to affect migraine sufferers adversely, so keep that in mind when considering birth control options.

As for acne? During a normal (i.e., non-Pill-related) menstrual cycle, the ovaries start producing progesterone at ovulation, which revs up the sebaceous glands. This results in more oil, oilier skin, and, you guessed it, pimples.

During the premenstrual time, woman tend to have more nightmares, as well as the type of sex dreams that make you blush the next morning.

The need to urinate frequently during one's period can be caused by fibroids, interstitial cystitis, or a urinary tract infection brought on by (we hate to say it) not changing one's pad often enough. After all, that pad is efficiently absorbing not only one's blood, but one's anal cooties, as well. One's period can also bring on marked fatigue, brought on by not only blood loss and the subsequent dip in iron levels, but by disturbed sleep. More than 70 percent of all women complain of sleep problems during their period, when hormone levels are at their lowest.

Believe it or not, one's menstrual cycle also seems to affect the kind of dreams one has. During the premenstrual time, women tend to have more nightmares, the kind that reflect fear of death and mutilation, as well as the type of sex dreams that make you blush the next morning.

Alcohol tolerance also varies depending on where one is in one's cycle. Unlike men, who seem capable of absorbing the same amount of beer no matter what time of the month it is, women clearly fluctuate: they seem to hold their liquor the best during their flow, the worst in the week before.

It's also been reported that all of a woman's senses are more acute during ovulation—for example, women tend to be more sensitive to smells, faint light, nuances in taste, even touch. One can mull over the possible biological advantages of this: might this possibly be related to an unconscious drive to find the right mate or initiate sex?

It's also been reported that during ovulation, women feel pretty damn good about themselves. This is the time when they generally feel the greatest sense of confidence and self-esteem, and are the most competitive, as well. Compare this to the premenstrual time, when women overwhelmingly feel not only pessimistic and self-hating, but even downright hostile to others.

For years, popular myth held that a woman's cycle was influenced by the moon and the tides.

We feel it should come as a relief to most women that symptoms, quirks, and moods as diverse as an insatiable craving for chocolate cupcakes, a sunny outlook, a raging migraine, or even a disturbingly erotic dream about that guy who works at the deli can all be linked somehow to the menstrual cycle. After all, menstruation is not just a 365-day-a-year process for all females between the onset of menarche and the end of menopause; it clearly wields a wide if mysterious influence over many far-flung aspects of our lives in ways we've only just begun to grasp.

Even though we all operate under the same basic physiological rules of menstruation, every woman's experience of her cycle is unique. A woman's period—the pain she suffers, her perception of that pain, the flow she has, the regularity of her cycle—is affected by numerous factors: her genes, her biochemical makeup, her weight (either losing or gaining too much weight can temporarily halt one's flow), even her personality and culture. For years, popular myth held that a woman's cycle was also influenced by the moon and the tides. More recently, however, that notion has been displaced by a more scientific theory—that a profound influence on a woman's menstrual cycle may in fact be no farther away than the people around her.

In 1971, a Harvard graduate student named Martha McClintock wrote an article in *Nature* magazine about something she had been pondering since her days at the women's college Wellesley: a notion she termed "menstrual synchrony." Her theory was that the menstrual cycles of women who live together in all-female environments, such as in prison, a convent, or a single-sex dorm, tend to synchronize over time. After studying 135 women who lived in the same college dorm and comparing them with women who didn't cohabit, she came up with a revolutionary proposal. Her theory was that not only did women's periods in fact line up with each other over time, but that it was all somehow triggered by pheromones—those potent yet odorless chemicals that are somehow thought to trigger responses in others unconsciously, through the sense of smell.

McClintock's theory instantly garnered a wild amount of attention, among both scientists and laypeople. Could it be true? Women began trading anecdotes about their own experiences and observations and how, sure enough, they could swear that all the toilets in their dorms clogged up at the same time due to the sudden overload of flushable tampons.

Yet subsequent studies of menstrual synchrony conducted by other researchers were, to put it mildly, consistently inconsistent. While sixteen studies confirmed McClintock's findings, another ten found no statistically significant pattern of synchrony whatsoever among cohabiting groups of women. Some studies even found that women became less synchronized the longer they lived together.

Some researchers argued that women couldn't possibly synchronize, since women's cycles are such different lengths—after two or three months, they'd immediately fall out of line with one another. Others, using basic math and probability, argued that since an average cycle is twenty-eight days, the maximum time between any two women getting their periods would be fourteen days, the minimum zero. This means the average difference would be a mere seven days. Anything less than seven days could then be argued to resemble synchrony, especially among such a relatively small group of women . . . even though it might be, of course, totally random.

Yet McClintock not only stuck to her guns, she continued to refine her argument. In 1998, she coauthored another article in *Nature* in which she reported on experiments that focused specifically on the possible effect of pheromones on menstruation. Cotton swabs were dabbed with armpit sweat taken from women during different points in their cycles. The swabs, by now liberally laced with the donors' pheromones, were then wiped on the sterilized upper lips of other women.

Before the whole idea makes you keel over in a dead faint, keep in mind that the women who were swabbed said that they honestly didn't smell anything . . . which would make sense, considering that that's how those sneaky pheromones work. And interestingly enough, the swabs did seem to have an effect on the length of the wipee's cycles, but not in a definite or consistent way. Instead, women's cycles were either shortened or lengthened, depending on how early in the donor's cycle the swab was taken.

So what is one to make of this research? If this is true, it seems to indicate that unconscious signals about the menstrual cycle are in fact constantly transmitted from woman to woman via pheromones, but in a shifting and cyclical way. If so, McClintock suggests that perhaps menstrual synchrony, or at least menstrual influence, can be seen in a social instead of an isolated context—that by influencing patterns of fertility, conception, and birth, it can serve to maximize, say, the chances of survival of the young in a given community. And furthermore, Natalie Angier points out that it's not just other women who seem to affect our cycles via those odorless messengers, the pheromones—it's men, as well.

Since it's documented that a woman who cohabits with a man tends to cycle more regularly than one who lives alone, wouldn't it make sense that she's in fact being influenced by his pheromones—the ones constantly wafting invisibly from his neck, his groin, his armpits? Is it just because of the typical height difference that so many of us straight women tend to enjoy nuzzling our guys in the neck, or are we simply trying in an unconscious way to get a good dose of his chemical messages? Certainly, it can be argued that a regular menstrual cycle favors conception. Are we in fact blindly in search of chemical triggers that will shore up our chances at propagation?

Normal, healthy menstruation is clearly still a mysterious terrain, rarely studied in any significant, well-funded way by any scientific institution or research lab . . . but why? Because it's so common as to be perceived as boring and inconsequential, at least to male researchers? It's only in its pathological state that doctors and scientists tend to sit up and take notice . . . in other words, when routinely good periods go bad.

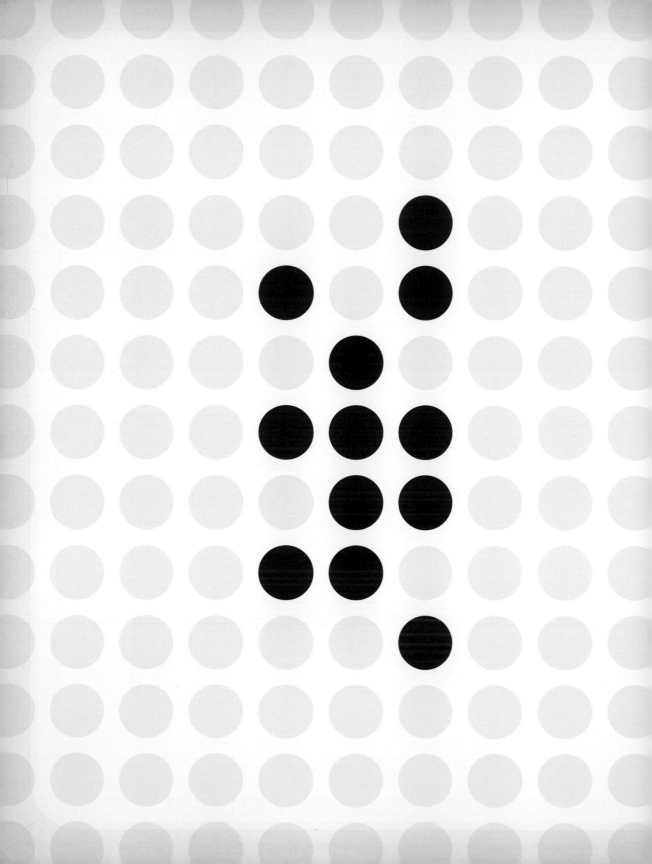

Chapter 12

WHEN GOOD PERIODS GO BAD

WE ARE NOT WHAT YOU'D CALL ESPECIALLY ghoulish or morbid. When finding ourselves in places such as, say, the Mutter Museum of anatomical oddities and pathological specimens in Philadelphia (home of preserved conjoined twins in a jar, a five-foot-long human colon, and the world's largest ovarian cyst), we tend to grow pale and feel an urgent need to be elsewhere. Nevertheless, we harbor a secret, sneaking fascination with that rarest of conditions, the oddest of medical oddities: vicarious menstruation.

Vicarious menstruation is a genuinely weird physical condition in which monthly bleeding occurs from parts of the female body . . . that aren't the uterus! This is not to be confused with stigmata, the inexplicable appearance of cuts and sores on the hands, feet, and sides of certain saints and martyrs, corresponding to the Five Wounds of Christ. Vicarious menstruation happens well outside the realm of religious mysticism, and is in fact related to the menstrual cycle. Once a month, blood painlessly, eerily flows for a few days from the lungs, breasts, fingers, elbows, mouth, ears, or even eyes, and then mysteriously stops.

Talk about embarrassing!

The organ most implicated in vicarious menstruation is the nose. One typical case, reported in 1908, involved a fifteen-year-old girl who bled heavily from her nose every month. The doctor "plugged the nares with absorbent cotton" and then prescribed regular dosings of the herb apocynum. Plugging those nares apparently did the trick, as the doctor triumphantly reported several months later that his patient had grown "lazy, fat and saucy, with normal menstruation."

Feeling a bit saucy ourselves, we would like to point out that bleeding from the nares, or nostrils, every month isn't as totally out there as it might first appear to the uninitiated. In fact, mucous membrane normally tends to be pretty responsive to estrogen, leading to the observation that many women routinely experience pronounced rhinorrhea before their periods. Rhinorrhea, which admittedly sounds as if one has begun to resemble a large, horned African mammal, is in fact plain old nasal swelling and congestion; and believe it or not, it's so common, it's considered a routine symptom of PMS.

Another explanation of one kind of vicarious menstruation involves surgical error. During common procedures like cesarean section, fibroid removal, or episiotomy, tiny shards from the uterine lining can be inadvertently implanted in the incision. Instead of peacefully dying, these bits of living tissue, pieces from one's own uterus, can on occasion settle down in their new home and even flourish. Next thing you know, they're acting as if it's business as usual, continuing to menstruate each month, as they respond to the ebb and flow of hormones.

Vicarious menstruation is one of those *Ripley's Believe It or Not* events that's good to trot out during long car rides or boring dinner parties. While few women actually experience it, this is by no means to say that there aren't all kinds of things that can and often do go wrong with menstruation. Some menstrual problems are mildly annoying, whereas others are extremely painful, messy, and downright dangerous. Some problems are as common as dirt, and others can even kill you. And still others, it can be argued, have changed history.

England's Queen Mary the First (funnily enough, nicknamed "Bloody Mary" for the way she went after those pesky Protestants) never menstruated and was technically barren. Without a male heir, the throne eventually went to her half sister, Elizabeth—thereby changing the history of England forever. Visionary French heroine and eventual saint Joan of Arc died at twenty, without ever having had a period. Feminist/anarchist Emma Goldman had a lifetime of painful menstruation, and experienced what appears to have been stress-induced premature menarche, fleeing the pogroms by swimming through icy waters. Were these women warriors affected by menstrual pathologies? We'll obviously never know . . . but it's an interesting new lens through which to view history, no?

One of the most typical menstrual problems is when women of reproductive age just stop menstruating altogether, or don't even start in the first place. This is called amenorrhea and can be caused by any number of routine and benign factors, such as pregnancy or breast-feeding. It can also be caused by pseudocyesis, or "hysterical pregnancy." This occurs when a woman is so absolutely convinced she's pregnant, she can literally go for years without having a period—and some have.

Primary amenorrhea happens when an adolescent female still hasn't started to menstruate, long after her peers have started skulking off to the bathroom during math class. And for those of you with searing memories of not getting your period until you were fourteen, fifteen, even sixteen, you can stop worrying: you definitely did *not* have pri-mary amenorrhea. Medically, "normal" is anywhere between nine and seventeen. It's only after a female hits eighteen sans period that she's said to have primary amenorrhea.

Primary amenorrhea can be caused by an underlying developmental problem brought on by severe stress or malnutrition. Funnily enough, it can be triggered by not only extreme weight loss caused by anorexia or bulimia, but morbid obesity, as well. It can also be caused by an underlying physiological condition, such as malfunctioning ovaries, the lack of a uterus, or some other genetic abnormality. In fact, many women with primary amenorrhea actually have an undiagnosed form of hermaphroditism that can be treated, once it's been detected.

Secondary amenorrhea occurs when a woman of reproductive age simply stops menstruating. The exact causes are still somewhat up in the air, although it seems to be triggered by hormonal imbalances, as well as by loss of weight and body fat. Amenorrhea can be brought on by rigorous athletic training or extreme dieting and, as a result, frequently affects athletes, models, ballet dancers, and women with eating disorders. Scarily, years of not menstruating can lead to significant bone loss and bone mineral density, especially in the lower spine.

But how does it work, anyway? What's the correlation between weight loss, athletic endeavor, and no periods?

To figure it out, let's first take out our calculators for our favorite piece of math trivia. When a woman loses 10 to 15 percent of her overall weight, she's actually losing up to *one-third* of her body fat. That, my friends, is a lot of fat! One theory suggests that since estrogen isn't just produced by the ovaries and adrenal glands, but by fatty tissue, such a drop in fat levels would mean a drop in one's estrogen levels, as well . . . causing menstruation to stop.

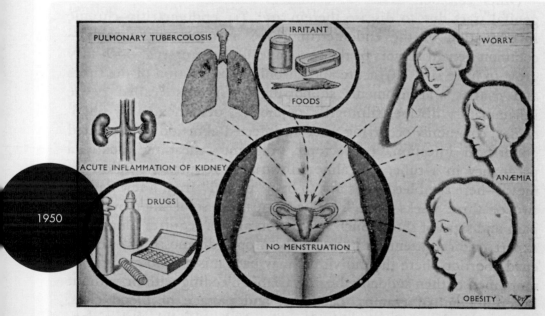

1950

FIG. 59—Eight pictures linked in one plate. Showing *no menstruation* in woman; its 7 causes illustrated.

Illustrated Encyclopedia of Sex, Cadillac Publishing Company

At the same time, there's evidence that amenorrhea among female athletes isn't just about fat levels. It could be that the production of endorphins, the naturally occurring "happy drug" the brain produces after intense exercise, somehow inhibits luteinizing hormone production up in the pituitary gland. Or it might instead have something to do with stress—not just the physical type, but the kind brought on by the intense focus and competition of serious sports. Some researchers make a convincing argument that emotional stress appears to be a predisposing factor for most cases of not just amenorrhea, but other kinds of menstrual disorders, as well, whether you're a serious athlete in training or just a regular ol' slug-a-bed, like the rest of us.

Fibroids occur in anywhere from 20 to 40 percent of all menstruating women, although most of us aren't even aware that they're there.

The flip side of amenorrhea is "menorrhagia," or excessive menstrual flow. Since average flow is anywhere up to six or so tablespoons' worth, anything more than that, or a flow that lasts longer than seven days, may indicate a problem. Menorrhagia is pretty common among IUD users. "Metrorrhagia" means bleeding outside of the normal time of one's cycle. Both metrorrhagia and menorrhagia can be caused by any one of a number of factors, benign or distinctly unfriendly—fibroids, cervical polyps, endometriosis, even heart disease—and should be checked out by one's doctor.

About one-fifth of all cases of irregular menstruation in women under forty are due to pelvic inflammatory disease, or, more snappily, PID. PID occurs when an infection contracted in, say, the vagina travels upward to the fallopian tubes and then up into the abdominal cavity. PID not only causes weird patterns of bleeding, it can be incredibly painful, dangerous, and potentially deadly. Luckily, it can be handled with antibiotics, although treatment often takes time.

There are other common causes for crazy, out-of-control menstrual flow. Myomas are a kind of tumor, and the most common are benign uterine fibroids. Fibroids occur in anywhere from 20 to 40 percent of all menstruating women, although most of us aren't even aware that they're there. No one seems to be exactly sure where they come from, although they seem to run in families. In addition, African-American women seem more prone to fibroids than other women.

While fibroids aren't caused by the menstrual cycle, their growth is stimulated by estrogen . . . and take it from us, boy, can they grow! The largest one in recorded history topped out at 143 pounds back in 1888. Needless to say, fibroids can be amazingly uncomfortable and also cause heavy bleeding for days on end. A woman can even start hemorrhaging and eventually develop anemia, in which case a doctor may very well recommend dilation and curettage, more commonly called a D&C. In a D&C, the cervix is dilated, or opened up; then a curette, a long rod with a sharp loop at the end, is inserted and used to carefully scrape out the lining of the uterus. A D&C requires general anesthesia if one is undergoing it or, in our case, even describing it. A woman may also opt for surgical removal of the fibroids or having the entire endometrium cauterized.

One thing to keep in mind: as far as some health-care providers are concerned, menstrual flow abnormalities are just a part of life for certain women. Certainly, once you hit your forties all bets are off: by then, most women normally experience heavier flow and wildly irregular cycles. Unless the problem itself poses an actual health threat or seems to indicate a bigger underlying problem, some doctors won't even prescribe treatment. They will instead suggest one merely hang tough until it all ends, i.e., menopause. While this may work fine for some women, it's just not an option for others. Furthermore, this doesn't mean you shouldn't seek out medical advice if you find you're mysteriously bleeding like a stuck pig for days on end.

There's a depressing fact that we ourselves never enjoy thinking about, which is that excessive or unusual bleeding can also be a sign of cancer. If you haven't already, please do everyone a favor and start getting in the habit of scheduling that regular Pap test! Not to sound like your mother or anything, but getting checked regularly for cervical cancer has got to be at least as important as having one's teeth examined, taxes filed, or winter woollies dry-cleaned.

Scientists have known for more than a hundred years that there's also a correlation between menstruation and epilepsy; studies have shown that seizures occur in 72 percent of females with epilepsy when they're bleeding. The most notorious of menstruating epileptics may well have been Massachusetts spinster/crazed ax murderess Lizzie Borden, made famous by the annoyingly catchy rhyme:

> Lizzie Borden took an ax
> And gave her mother forty whacks
> And when she saw what she had done
> She gave her father forty-one.

In fact, thirty-three-year-old Lizzie probably suffered from epilepsy of the temporal lobe, only had seizures when she was having her period, and most likely did kill both her father and stepmother during one such crazed menstrual bout. This is not to make Lizzie appear to be some kind of hapless victim of her uterus; there seemed to be quite a few unresolved hostility issues in the Borden household to begin with, as evidenced by at least one previous murder attempt. Nevertheless, Lizzie was acquitted of all charges, due to a combination of inept police work, flabby prosecution, and the overriding disbelief in 1892 that a nice girl could do such an awful thing. Lizzie's seizures eventually stopped when she hit menopause: a happy ending for Lizzie, if not for her parents.

Menstruation can routinely aggravate various chronic illnesses and disorders, causing flare-ups and outbreaks: migraines, insomnia, asthma, arthritis. These almost always die down again once flow is over. During one's period, chronic infections like shingles or herpes are more likely to rouse themselves from dormancy and make an unwelcome appearance; diabetics find they have a harder time controlling their condition. And during the premenstrual time, all kinds of diseases, like pneumonia, hepatitis, scarlet fever, and the flu, tend to occur more frequently.

"And what about all that blood loss?" we hear you ask. What about anemia, the specter of which has been used to terrify girls into eating disgusting platefuls of liver and other organ meats since time immemorial? What about leaching all that precious iron, month after month, year after year?

Believe it or not, a normal, healthy woman doesn't need a whole lot of extra iron to replace what she loses during menstruation; as a matter of fact, 90 percent is automatically replenished by one's body. Nevertheless, women do regularly lose twice as much iron as do men, and therefore, a passing nod to replacing it is in order. Some find iron supplements a tad binding, so dietary iron is always a worthwhile alternative. Good sources are meat, poultry, and fish if one eats such things and green, leafy vegetables, enriched grains, and dried fruits if one doesn't. And since iron absorption seems to be influenced by other dietary factors, it always helps to eat a balanced diet, especially one that contains a lot of vitamin C.

Overwhelmingly, the single most common menstrual problem women suffer from is endometriosis, a disease that is both caused and aggravated by menstruation

Endometriosis is much more likely to occur in women who have never been pregnant, and has thus been named "the career woman's disease."

(although postmenopausal women suffer from it, as well). Here's the deal: in a healthy woman, endometrial tissue is found only in the uterus. Occasionally, however, tiny bits of endometrial tissue or clumps of cells can be carried out of the uterus and into the pelvic cavity by one's menstrual flow.

This isn't such a big deal on its own, and in most cases, a woman's immune system is able to handily dispose of any stray cells floating around. For others, however, should any of those fragments or cells come into contact with scarred or injured tissue, woe is you! They will happily attach themselves to their new home and immediately commence to reproduce. Those little devils can set up shop on the diaphragm, fallopian tubes, ovaries, bladder, or intestines, or inside the abdominal cavity. These endometrial colonies grow and grow, and as they respond to the hormonal cycle, they continue to act as if they were still in the uterus, doing what they're programmed to do: thickening and building up when exposed to estrogen, then bleeding when estrogen levels drop. This cycle eventually causes scarring wherever the colonies have landed, as well as the formation of cysts. Since it's a progressive disease, it ultimately leads to chronic discomfort, backache, nausea, and pain during sex and/or bowel movements. If left untreated, it can cause infertility in 30 to 40 percent of its victims and is one of the leading causes of childlessness worldwide.

More than 150 million women suffer from endometriosis worldwide, whether they're aware of it or not . . . and if you have a mother or sister with endometriosis, your risk is seven times greater. It's also much more likely to occur in women who have never been pregnant, and has thus been nicknamed "the career woman's disease." Ironically, the upswing in cases in the past few decades may well be due to social progress: as more women postpone maternity until their late twenties and early thirties, they're more vulnerable to this painful and often dangerous condition.

So what's a woman to do if she suffers from endometriosis? Or, for that matter, from severe dysmenorrhea, or fibroids? What are you supposed to do if your periods are genuinely screwing up your life?

Theoretically, one solution would be to just stay pregnant for the rest of your life, since pregnancy is a natural ovulation suppressant. So is breast-feeding, at least for a short while. During breast-feeding, one's body produces prolactin while inhibiting the release of gonadotrophin, which in turn blocks ovulation and menstruation. Unfortunately, as birth control, this method is at best 98 percent effective, and only for the those first few months after giving birth.

The two most common ways to treat severe menstrual problems are through drugs or medical procedures. Every woman has to weigh her options carefully, because what works for her may be totally unacceptable to another. Any course of treatment she wants to undertake will have to be one based not only on her doctor's diagnosis, the severity of the symptoms, and the possible risks of therapy, but on her own needs and concerns, as well.

There are chemical means of suppressing menstruation. These are generally contraceptives, synthetic hormones that can be administered orally, vaginally, via implant, or by injection. Taken regularly, they will regulate, reduce, or even eliminate one's menstrual flow altogether, and also bring marked relief to anyone suffering from regular, severe pain. While there appear to be health benefits associated with long-term hormone use, there are also notable risks, especially for women who are over thirty-five, smoke cigarettes, and/or are overweight.

To treat endometriosis surgically, a woman can opt for varying degrees of just how radical an approach she finds acceptable. She can get a D&C, but if it's not performed correctly, the procedure can result in infection, uterine perforation, or even infertility. Alternatively, a doctor can remove only the endometrial implants and leave everything else alone. Another option is for the entire endometrium to be cauterized, in a procedure called endometrial resection or ablation. These methods are considered fairly conservative, surgically speaking, although there's a possibility that the endometrium or the implants could grow back. And like all medical procedures, there are always risks and possible complications that should be weighed seriously.

Myomectomy, in which the fibroids are removed hysteroscopically, through a tube, isn't even considered surgery and can be done in a doctor's office. One's doctor, however, may argue against it, since it does take a certain amount of skill and experience; it definitely pays to find out how many he or she has performed to date. One will also probably be told that her fibroids could grow back. This, however, isn't necessarily the worst-case scenario; even if a woman tends to grow fibroids like dandelions in the springtime, most don't cause any problems at all.

The most radical way to stop menstruation and all of its problems is via hysterectomy, i.e., the surgical removal of the uterus. The removal of the ovaries is called an oophorectomy, and the two procedures are often performed together.

The first recorded hysterectomy was done in ancient Greece, in A.D. 100, and it was performed through the vagina. As doctors since time immemorial believed that the uterus was the seat of everything wrong with a woman, untold millions of healthy organs have been removed over the centuries, regardless of any proof that the operation did anything other than kill a whole lot of women; by the late 1880s, there was a 50 percent death rate for the procedure.

And what are the effects of hysterectomy, anyway? To us, they seem wildly contradictory. Regarding sex, for instance, some women report the loss of pleasurable uterine contractions during orgasm, diminished lubrication, and pain caused by scar tissue in the vagina. Yet other women are delighted by the freedom from uterine cramps and pain, as well as the relief of never having to worry about getting pregnant again. For them, having a hysterectomy is a shot in the arm and a huge boost to their sex lives. Some women suffer from depression after having the uterus removed, whereas others report being much happier. Some women (virtually all heterosexual) worry that their femininity and allure have diminished after their hysterectomy; still others feel an upsurge in confidence.

These, clearly, are intensely personal reactions that are hard to predict. After all, who can really say how anyone would react to the surgical removal of an organ, especially one so closely tied to our gender as the good old uterus?

Moreover, there are also significant physical complications worth weighing if one is seriously contemplating a hysterectomy. After all, it *is* major abdominal surgery, with all of the usual risks (adhesions, lesions, intestinal blockage, thrombosis). There are other possible complications worth weighing, as well. Even if one has opted to keep one's ovaries, for example, they occasionally end up inert. Furthermore, the sudden absence of the prostaglandins normally produced by the uterus may increase one's risk of heart disease and high blood pressure.

Scarily enough, some women don't realize until too late that what they *thought* was a plain old hysterectomy also involved an oophorectomy, as well . . . and that the surgical removal of their ovaries brings on a sudden drop in hormones that can bring about other problems. Such possible side effects may include arthritis, osteoporosis, chronic fatigue, greater susceptibility to heart disease, depression, and mood disorders. Oophorectomy before menopause can also put a woman at greater risk for dementia and Parkinson's disease. And who needs that, we ask?

For virtually all of history, the uterus has been pretty much thought of as either a wandering kind of animal, a passive sack that a baby grew in once in a while, or the seat of a woman's emotions. But in fact, we now know it produces hormones, proteins, and sugars, not to mention prostaglandins that help our vascular tone and possibly help keep our circulatory system in good health. The uterus is also a crazy drug factory, making and secreting huge amounts of natural opiates that are closely related to marijuana, heroin, and morphine (we'd probably all be in prison if anyone in the White House knew). It's an extraordinarily complex organ, as mysterious as the bottom of the sea, that clearly has a dynamic yet still unknown relationship with the rest of the body . . . and it's not something to be snipped out and disposed of lightly.

And yet the United States is currently one of the world's leaders in the procedure; every year, more than 600,000 women have a hysterectomy, making it the second most commonly performed surgery in the country. (Hey, and do you know what the *first* most commonly performed procedure is? A hint: it involves the same organ, the only organ, in fact, that doesn't have an analogous equivalent in the male anatomy. Answer: the cesarean section.)

This translates to the fact that the uterus of at least one out of three American women, mostly between the ages of twenty and forty-nine, will be surgically removed, and often the ovaries and cervix, as well. Overwhelmingly, the surgery is performed for noncancerous problems: fibroids, endometriosis, benign growths, uterine prolapse, menorrhagia. Disturbingly, there are some weird discrepancies in who gets the procedure and who doesn't. Rates are twice as high in the South as they are in the Northeast, and higher in rural areas than in cities. African-American women in their early forties have the highest hysterectomy rate of all. And what's most disturbing is that some researchers believe that at least a third of all hysterectomies are medically unnecessary.

THE COST OF BEING FEMALE

Have you ever wondered, as did wild-eyed feminists in the 1970s, if there's something wrong about our even having to pay for fem-care products in the first place? Gloria Steinem once quipped, "If men could menstruate...sanitary supplies would be federally funded and free," just like the toilet paper and soap in any public restroom. And why is it that in many states in the United States, not to mention countries like Canada and Australia, tampons and pads aren't considered "nonluxury" items, i.e., essential, and are thus subject to sales tax? Do you really consider that monthly packet of plugs a luxury?

As we've said before, we know that menstruation is one of our most personal processes and that the perception of pain is wildly subjective. Medical and surgical solutions to menstrual problems have unquestionably helped untold numbers of women live happier, fuller lives; what's more, we fully support any female's right to control her own body.

That being said—we're still fans of the uterus. What can we say? As Natalie Angier pointed out so eloquently in her book *Woman: An Intimate Geography*, "To make a truly informed choice, we need information." If you're being driven to despair by menstruation, get all the facts you can and think twice.

And then sleep on your decision and think again.

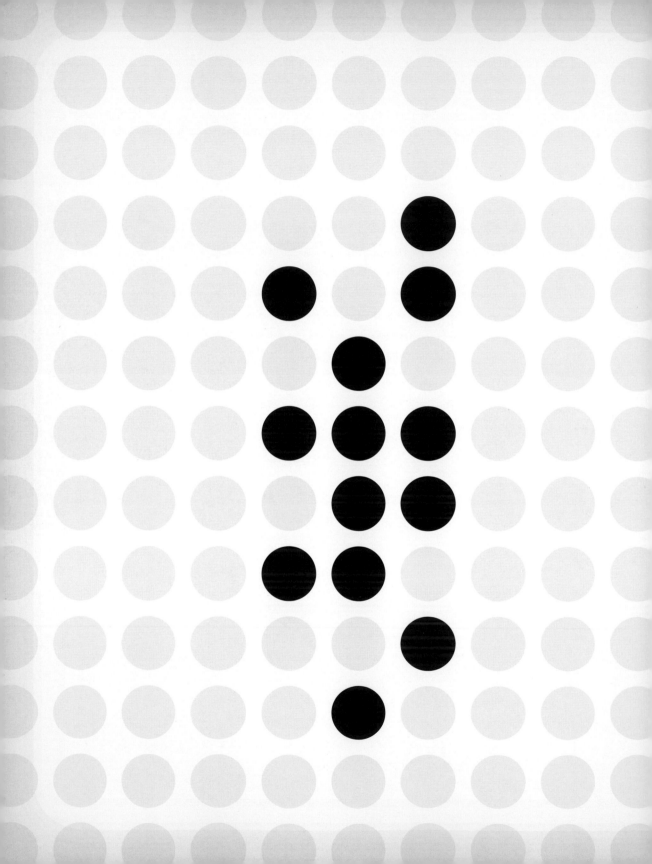

Chapter 13

HEY, IS IT GETTING HOT IN HERE?

WOULD YOU EVER PAY MONEY TO SWALLOW horse urine?

Okay . . . that's kind of a disgusting question to ask out of the blue, and we're sorry we just sort of sprang it on you. That being said, we feel compelled to ask this because, believe it or not, one of the bestselling prescription meds *of all time* is created using that selfsame liquid.

Premarin—introduced by Wyeth-Ayerst in 1943 to alleviate symptoms of menopause—is a synthetic estrogen product extracted from pregnant mares' urine (PMU). Currently, more than nine million women in the United States take it for estrogen replacement therapy; according to the Humane Society of the United States, it takes about fifty thousand not-very-well-treated horses kept pregnant as continuously as possible on more than five hundred "PMU farms." The foals are prematurely weaned and a lucky few are auctioned off to private owners. The rest are fattened up at feedlots

"PREMARIN"

1955

the choice of thousands of physicians for estrogen replacement therapy

Wyeth

until they're big enough to be slaughtered for their meat. And all this is just to keep the labs stocked with enough pregnant mares' urine to meet the increasing demand.

Pardon us . . . but *blechh*.

One might reasonably think, *Well, if any of those women actually knew what was in it, they'd stop taking it, wouldn't they?* But in (creepy) fact, even that unsavory piece of information probably wouldn't make any difference at all, and the reason is simple.

We women fear aging. All people do, but it's worse for women, even worse for American women, and even worse still, at least according to one study, if one is straight rather than gay. As smart and tough and accomplished a cookie as she might be, the average woman is trained from the moment she turns thirty to start dreading those telltale signs: the chin swags, the odd hair growing out of a mole, the crow's-feet, the thickening waist, the thinning hair.

And many of us are terrified of menopause. We fear becoming a lampoonable cartoon of a woman with ludicrous symptoms: hot flashes, temper tantrums, night sweats. We dread turning into a lumpish, sexless gnome in a pastel sweatsuit, existing solely for the free cheese samples at the supermarket and owning too many mugs with funny sayings on them. And even if we don't have a maternal bone in our body, we brood endlessly about the last gasp of fertility, the end of our "usefulness" as women.

But where does this unholy terror come from? Good question, we reply . . . and suggest, as is so often the case when it comes to menstruation, that we take a good look back through the annals of history for a possible explanation.

For centuries, menopause wasn't seen as a natural function, but instead as something gone seriously wrong, an actual disease. It's important to remember that before the twentieth century, just the idea of women routinely living a third of their lives after menopause was beyond freakish. Today, while the age of menopause hasn't changed, life expectancy for the average American woman has ballooned: from forty-nine in 1900 to nearly eighty-one in 2007. As a result, there are close to fifty million midlife women living in the United States today. Yet until quite recently in world history, a woman living past her childbearing years was like a total eclipse of the sun, a rare anomaly to be viewed with suspicion, even fear.

In the Middle Ages, witchcraft was considered a reasonable explanation for the sudden stoppage of blood. Even before that, women who stopped menstruating were assumed to be out of balance somehow. From the 1921 book *Menstruation and Its Disorders:* "By the old school of humoral pathologists, the cessation of menstruation was looked upon as a matter of serious consequence, often causing serious disorders and calling for the operation of blood-letting. Perhaps these old observers are in part responsible for the great dread with which the menopause is even now looked forward to by a large proportion of womankind."

This, of course, was a not-so-veiled reference to Hippocrates and his wacky but popular "humorism" theory. As bloodletting mimicked menstruation, it was thus considered a cure for the disease of menopause. Leeches were routinely applied to a woman's back, neck, and genitalia—all to get that stagnating, diseased blood out.

It took the original Freudian, Sigmund himself, to arguably move the entire discussion about menopause one eensy-weensy baby step forward by deciding it was a neurotic condition rather than a clinical disease. In his opinion, menopausal women were "quarrelsome, peevish, and argumentative, petty and miserly." He heartily recommended the liberal use of drugs, namely sedatives, to keep menopausal women calm and collected.

Thanks to Freud, equating menopause with mental illness became a given. Yet even insanity wasn't considered the worst part about menopause. On a planet where for thousands of years, even today, a woman's worth has been judged exclusively by the productivity of her womb, what the hell was the point of a barren woman, anyway? What's more, the menopausal female was no longer considered any good for sex, either. In 1913, T. W. Shannon, the author of *Self Knowledge*, wrote that a husband "should have no sexual relations during the change of life in his wife. If the husband wishes to protect the health of his wife and himself, prolong their lives, increase their usefulness and happiness he must bring himself to complete self-control"; and what's more, that sex during menopause was both unsanitary and unhygienic, as it would most likely cause the buzz kill known as "flooding," a veritable deluge of menstrual blood.

All this talk about sexual relations was, of course, assuming a man even wanted to get anywhere near his perimenopausal wife. Even this was questionable, especially if he was unfortunate to have read such descriptions of her decay in the 1954 *Illustrated Encyclopedia of Sex:* "The layer of fat in the region of the mons veneris and in the large lips of the vulva starts to shrink. The vulva becomes smaller and flabbier, the small lips become withered and change into thin folds. The fatty glands, formerly present in more than adequate amounts, disappear almost completely, so that there are only remnants of them left."

Similarly, Emil Novak, in his 1921 book, *Menstruation and Its Disorders,* dutifully reports that "the vulva loses its velvety vascular appearance and becomes thin, pale, and transparent looking, giving the surface a rather pasty appearance," and makes sure to mention that pubic hair becomes "gray and straggly." Helpfully contributing to the positive tone, *The Illustrated Encyclopedia of Sex* describes in detail how the loss of skin's elasticity keeps it from being able to hold fat deposits in place, so that the womanly curves men find so attractive "literally slide down, and that, in particular, the cheeks, throat, breasts, abdomen, hips and buttocks become flabby, distorting the body."

It's true that in a time when women had nothing, really, except their families, the loss of fertility plus

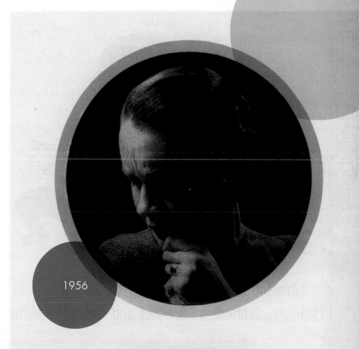

their grown children's independence often combined to create emotional stress and a sense of worthlessness that peaked just as menopause was starting. The resulting combination was probably enough to make any reasonable female seem neurotic, depressed, even a little unhinged on occasion.

There was in addition the genuine fear that menopause could cause serious disease. Hippocrates himself wrote that menopausal women "are frequently affected with the itch, the elephantiasis, boils, erysipelatous disorders, or scirrhous cancerous disease."

Don't let the fancy-pants, old Greek medical language throw you. He was, in fact, talking about cancer. Considering that abnormal bleeding is a known symptom of uterine cancer, dramatic menstrual changes probably convinced many women in years past they were at death's door. No wonder countless women dreaded getting older and the terrifying physical, emotional, sexual, and social changes that went along with it.

Yet is the end of menstruation really that awful? So bad that today, we've been reduced to quaffing en masse what sounds like a witch's brew of horse pee in a frantic attempt to stave off the inevitable? What exactly *is* menopause, anyway?

First off, menopause is actually something that isn't: namely, it's the absence of menstrual flow for twelve consecutive months. The seemingly endless changes leading up to it, with all of those familiar symptoms, aren't actually menopause at all, but perimenopause ("peri" meaning "around" or "near"), and that can last for up to fifteen years. Out of an average reproductive life of thirty-seven years or so, perimenopause can comprise quite a significant chunk.

No one's quite sure exactly what kicks off the entire process, and while the average age is fifty-one, all kinds of factors (smoking, drinking, radiation treatment or chemotherapy, removal of the ovaries and/or uterus, family history) can bring about an earlier start. On the other hand, women who are heavier, married, or have never had children seem to start somewhat later, as do women who suffer from uterine fibroids.

Perimenopause can often begin in one's thirties and be the silent, undiagnosed reason for all kinds of annoying physical and emotional changes going on. The process can take such a long time, women and their health-care providers often miss the most obvious (or not so obvious) explanation: that it's actually hormonal shifts that are causing all those mysterious headaches, backaches, sleep problems, skin eruptions, and mood swings.

Menopause isn't directly related to menarche. Nevertheless, many women ruefully call it menarche in reverse, as it's a similar gradual shift in hormones, albeit in the opposite direction, and one often fraught with similar physical and emotional turmoil, as well. In fact, many of the symptoms are eerily similar to what we went through as adolescents, during our early days of menstruation. What adult woman ever thinks she'll have to deal with irregular cycles, unexpected leaks, acne breakouts, and off-the-wall mood swings all over again?

Most women go through menopause in their late forties or early fifties. Still others stop menstruating permanently in their thirties or even twenties, in which case it's known as premature menopause or premature ovarian failure. Younger women then have to grapple with the fact that their ability to reproduce is gone, often before they've had time to have children or even decide whether they wanted any. They also suffer an increased risk for heart disease and osteoporosis, against which estrogen acts as effective protection.

Menopause doesn't refer to the years after your period ends. Once those twelve period-free months have passed, you're technically postmenopausal. It's not a disease, nor is it the end of your life, not by a long shot. Given current longevity rates, the average postmenopausal woman can look forward to a good thirty years of life left . . . which, funnily enough, is just about as long as she was menstrual in the first place. It's a natural and inevitable process that will, most assuredly, happen to any woman at some point or another. Yet from all the hubbub surrounding the subject, menopause has apparently morphed into something practically worse than death itself. The medical and pharmaceutical companies share more than part of the blame, continuing to encourage our fears by pushing treatments that have often proved to be more questionable, dangerous, or nauseating than previously realized.

During perimenopause, the reproductive system gradually shuts down. Ovaries stop responding to stimulating hormones sent from the brain, which leads to diminished egg maturation. This leads to decreased estrogen and progesterone production, which eventually throws the entire reproductive system into a mild tizzy. While the process is natural and actually relatively simple, it can feel like the most confusing, out-of-control, and basically endless process one's body has ever gone through.

One of the first signs of perimenopause is irregular periods. Regardless of how much of a Swiss clock one's ovaries may have been for much of one's adult life, one may suddenly find oneself back in eighth grade, when cycles came and went at will, with unexpected torrents of blood coming out of nowhere, alternating with mere dribbles. For some perimenopausal women, cycles slow down and periods come further and further apart, even skipping a month or two altogether. For others, the reverse is true: as the ovaries stop releasing eggs and the accompanying hormones aren't secreted, the increasingly insistent pituitary gland sends out more and more stimulating hormones, trying to jump-start the cycle. Ovulation happens earlier, the whole cycle speeds up, and pretty soon, it may seem as if the second one damn period ends, another starts up almost immediately.

Clots and bleeding for fifteen days, bleed through two super-plus tampons, and a pad at night, only to wake up in bloody sheets or bleed through clothes at work, never knowing when it's coming.

—Jennifer B. (47)

Some women experience far lighter flow, others much heavier, and some women have periods that are so unnervingly intense, there's actual clotting involved. The four-day average is thrown out the window like last week's lunch: perimenopausal periods can last anywhere from a couple of days to a couple of weeks. Heavy periods can be brought on by excessive uterine buildup due to lowered progesterone levels. They can also be caused by fibroids, suffered by 40 percent of all perimenopausal women. And even though such symptoms usually go away by themselves after menopause, that can be cold comfort to many women.

Hands down, the superstar of perimenopausal symptoms, the one that literally needs no introduction, is the hot flash: the intense, pizza-oven-esque heat that usually starts in the waist or chest and rapidly zooms up to the neck, face, and scalp.

That internal inferno promptly unleashes a veritable blouse-soaking, hair-drenching sweat storm, as the body desperately tries to cool down . . . and that, in turn, leads to severe, all-over chills.

Not all women experience hot flashes, and even the ones who do have their own patterns. Hot flashes vary in intensity, frequency, and duration from person to person. Some women have dozens a day for years, while others have no more than a handful, total. Some hot flashes last for a few seconds, whereas others can go on for half an hour; the average is three to six minutes, although to some women, it can feel like an eternity.

Hot flashes aren't just an annoying way to ruin a silk blouse. They can also bring on nausea, dizziness, rapid heartbeat, and breathlessness, plus feelings of anxiety and suffocation. For one woman, hot flashes are a mild inconvenience; yet another may feel as if a severe panic attack is coming on, as her body is swamped in heat and she slowly starts to asphyxiate. The entire experience can be negligible, humiliating, nothing much, debilitating, mildly amusing, or horrifying.

[Hot flashes are] vicious, evil, all-consuming, demanding, unpredictable, hitting anywhere, anytime. When I am at home, I run to the fridge and stand in front of the freezer—I started wearing tanks so I could strip wherever I was. I hope those furnace-like outbursts of hormonal upheaval will never, never return.

—Carla S. (51)

Some women get a funny feeling, an aura or premonition that a hot flash is headed their way and can at least steel themselves for the inevitable; others just get blindsided by that wall of heat. While hot flashes seem to come out of nowhere, eating hot or spicy food, drinking alcohol or caffeine, or being stressed out can all be triggers. When they happen at night, they're

The worst of it are the night sweats! Covers on, covers off, legs in, legs out, clothes on, clothes off. I have not had a full eight hours of sleep in I don't know how long.

—Gerry C. (49)

called night sweats and can make one's normal sleep patterns totally wack, even leading to sleep deprivation. It's been reported that up to 75 percent of women experience night sweats at some point.

And yet menstrual disruptions and hot flashes are just two stars in the large cast of perimenopausal symptoms. Women routinely experience mood swings, spaciness, tearfulness, mental fogginess, and forgetfulness, making it a Herculean challenge to realize that the keys one has misplaced are actually in one's hand. There's often unexpected weight gain, and invariably in the last places one wants it, namely the hips, waist, and abdomen (although sometimes the breasts, as well). Speaking of breasts, they can often feel achey and tender to the point of actual pain.

That memory-loss thing is killing me. . . . I was a sharp person all my life and remembered most details, and now I don't remember anything.

—Samantha W. (55)

In addition, perimenopausal women may experience insomnia, dizziness, vertigo and/or migraines, heart palpitations, dry skin, hair loss, and urinary incontinence.

Another area of great concern to many, as well as to their partners, is sex. As they approach menopause, many women feel their libidos evaporate like morning dew on a hot day, whereas others feel an unprecedented surge of randiness. But regardless of interest level, thinning of the vaginal walls and less lubrication can make intercourse uncomfortable, even painful.

So here's the million-dollar question: knowing all this, what is the average middle-aged woman to do when told she doesn't have to go through the whole humiliating process? That menopause is

I think my main complaint is the declining sex drive. . . . Part of the problem is the fact that I feel like the Sahara desert down there. I want to have sex, but my body is not responding like it used to.

—Gail A. (49)

inherently unnatural and unnecessary, and that for the price of a prescription, she can do an easy end run around all the hot flashes, the night sweats, and libido loss, holding on to her youth and vitality until

she finally keels over at ninety? "Women will be emancipated only when the shackles of hormone deprivation are loosened!" "Menopause is completely preventable. No woman need suffer menopause or any of its symptoms if she receives preventative treatment before the onset of menopause!" Hearing such heady assurances, what forty-six-year-old wouldn't feel a flutter of hope stirring in her ever-drooping bosom?

And that's exactly how Dr. Robert A. Wilson, gynecologist and author of the bestselling 1966 book *Feminine Forever,* convinced so many women for years that long-term hormone replacement therapy (HRT) was the way to go. In the book's intro, Dr. Robert B. Greenblatt eloquently lauded the seemingly selfless author: "Like a gallant knight he has come to rescue his fair lady not at the time of her bloom and flowering but in her despairing years; at a time of life when the preservation and prolongation of her femaleness are so paramount."

In fact, scientists had been searching for hormones, or at least for the way the brain communicated chemically to the body, since the 1800s. And when synthetic hormones were first created in the 1930s, they were quickly marketed for a variety of female ailments and conditions, in utter disregard for any potential health hazards.

Freud himself may have inadvertently started the HRT ball rolling by suggesting all women should be sedated when their periods ended, but tranquilizers and anti-depressants were a mere bowl of Beer Nuts once hormone therapy rolled along. The medicalization of menopause provided drug companies with an opportunity that was practically as good as printing money. By convincing women that all they needed was synthetic estrogen to make up for failing ovaries, thus sidestepping the inevitable pitfalls of aging, pharmaceutical companies struck a veritable gold mine—preying on widespread fear and ignorance.

In the mid-twentieth century, drug manufacturers didn't have to prove a drug's effectiveness; they only had to show it wasn't inherently dangerous to the user. Nice that the FDA set the bar so high, wasn't it? By the mid-1960s, after Wyeth effectively sold gynecologists on the powers of Premarin as a rejuvenator and mood stabilizer, 12 percent of postmenopausal women were regularly taking estrogen supplements. And yet it wasn't until the publication of *Forever Feminine* in 1966 that HRT went solid gold.

In his book, Wilson makes an untold number of totally unsubstantiated statements (i.e., lies and threats), apparently the crazier the better, in order to convince women of the powers of HRT: "Instead of being condemned to witness the death of their own womanhood . . . they will remain fully feminine." "Women have the right to remain women. They shouldn't have to live as sexual neuters for half their lives." And why stop there? "Menopause is curable. . . . The bodily changes typical of middle age can be reversed and sexual function restored, along with a fully feminine appearance." Our personal favorite: "Many physicians simply refuse to recognize menopause for what it is—a serious, painful, and often crippling disease." Wilson goes on and on and on, including several weird, personal asides in which he shares his profound aversion for that current fashion trend, stretch pants.

We would like to be charitable and imagine Wilson to have been just the kind of guy his jacket blurb suggested: a chivalrous, Sean Connery–esque King Arthur out to rescue his beloved but aging Queen Guinevere from the horrors of decrepitude. But in fact, Wilson wasn't a disinterested nonparticipant in the HRT campaign. Although it was barely mentioned at the time and is nowhere to be found in the book, both his research and *Forever Feminine* were quietly funded by Wyeth, producers of Premarin.

Eventually, the FDA banned Wilson from certain research; yet thanks to him, enthusiastic support for HRT continued for years. Magazines like *Time* sang its praises; Dr. David Reuben concurred with Wilson's theories about menopausal women in his bestselling 1969 book, *Everything You Always Wanted to Know About Sex (But Were Afraid to Ask)*: "As the estrogen is shut off, a woman comes as close as she can to being a man. . . . To many women, the menopause marks the end of their useful life." As a result, estrogen sales went through the roof.

But the mares' urine hit the fan in 1975, when estrogen replacement therapy was linked with endometrial cancer. *The New England Journal of Medicine*, hardly a

At any age, you can be...
FEMININE FOREVER
by
ROBERT A. WILSON, M.D.
The documented story of one of modern medicine's most revolutionary developments and breakthroughs—the realization that menopause is a hormone deficiency and totally preventable. Now, almost every woman, regardless of age, can safely live a full sex life for her entire life.

1966

Pocket Bo

hotbed of medical hysteria, published disturbing reports showing that postmenopausal women taking estrogen supplements had *fourteen times* as much risk of developing endometrial cancer as women who didn't. Estrogen sales came to a screeching halt, and by 1979, it was only prescribed for treating hot flashes and vaginal dryness. As a medical supertrend, estrogen therapy appeared to be going the way of the Hula Hoop and the Pet Rock.

But because all good horror stories demand a third act, there was a plot twist yet to come. Doctors discovered that the hormone progestogen would counteract the cancer-inducing properties of estrogen. What a relief! It was hormone therapy with all the cancer-causing kinks taken out. To launch its retooled product in the 1980s, Wyeth put together a hugely expensive marketing campaign, and as a result, Prempro, its new estrogen/progestogen combo pill, became a bona fide hit.

For a while, the combination of estrogen and progestogen seemed to be just the ticket: not only did it alleviate menopause symptoms, but it also protected bones from osteoporosis. What's more, it was starting to look as if the hormone combo also prevented cardiac disease . . . happy news indeed for the Wyeth gang! By the 1990s, HRT for the postmenopausal woman was again a no-brainer, having successfully pulled itself back from the brink of medical obsolescence by again promising her she needn't fear becoming either "a dull-minded but sharp-tongued caricature of her former self" or "one of the saddest of human spectacles" (more quotes from Wilson's *Feminine Forever*).

And then, researchers finally got around to those long-term studies, to document HRT's effectiveness. It turned out that women who already had heart disease were more likely to have a heart attack if on estrogen therapy. And in 2002, the bomb dropped. Women's Health Initiative concluded that while HRT did have some health benefits—allaying osteoporosis and reducing the risk of colorectal cancer—these in no way outweighed the increased risk for blood clots, heart disease, stroke, and breast cancer.

Talk about a buzz kill. The National Institutes of Health abruptly ended the study, sending its sixteen thousand participants letters recommending they stop taking the drugs. The NIH sent out a press release in December, adding "steroidal estrogens" to its known carcinogen list, calling out estrogen in both replacement therapy and birth control pills as a potential cancer-causing agent.

And yet the HRT story still isn't over. Reluctant to relinquish such a dependable source of vast revenue, Wyeth introduced even lower-dose versions of Prempro for treating osteoporosis and postmenopausal symptoms in 2003. But in October 2007, a jury awarded a $134.5 million verdict to three Nevada women who argued that Premarin and Prempro were responsible for their breast cancer. There are currently over five thousand similar lawsuits in state and federal courts across the country.

In spite of the bad press and the stream of lawsuits, drug companies are still actively marketing their hormonal wares. These days, however, manufacturers market hormone therapy more realistically for short-term symptom relief than as a long-term elixir of dewy youth. And yet it's clear women are still being misled by assurances like the following from premarinonline.com: "PREMARIN can help guide you through this graceful transition. Because PREMARIN has been women's best friend for over 60 years and will always be." With friends like that, who needs asbestos?

Yet all is not lost for perimenopausal women. In her 2006 book, *The Wisdom of Menopause*, Dr. Christiane Northrup suggests that instead of limiting themselves to just prescription drugs from big pharma, perimenopausal women should also consider supplementing their dwindling hormone levels in alternative ways, such as with herbs and diet. She sings the praises of foods like soy and flaxseed, which are rich in the natural hormones found in plants, as well as certain berries and grains, which contain bioflavonoids.

More intriguing, Northrup also suggests that we ditch the whole one-size-fits-all way of thinking about hormone replacement. She advises working with one's physician and special pharmacists to develop an individualized hormone replacement plan made up of "bioidentical hormones," customized to one's own needs and symptoms.

Bioidentical hormones can't be patented, which means you won't be finding them manufactured by the big pharmaceuticals anytime soon. And long-term studies have yet to be conducted, so their safety over time remains an open question. That being said, they don't seem to have the same carcinogenic effect as Premarin or Prempro—

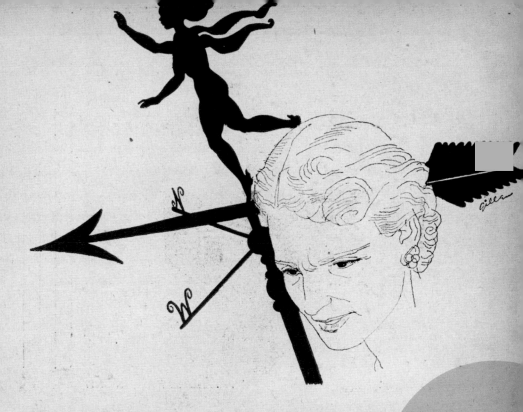

SUBJECT TO CHANGE WITHOUT NOTIC

You can assure women who seek to avoid
the nervous tension, emotional imbalance
and mental depression of the menopause that modern estrogenic therapy brings symptomatic relief in many
cases without undue pain or waste of time. When Abbott's Estrone
Aqueous Suspension is used, a few injections are sufficient in many
instances to keep the patient in comfort for weeks. Clinical experiments
have shown that out of 44 women who received three weekly treatments,
43 experienced relief for three to sixteen weeks.[1] As Estrone Aqueous
Suspension is prepared in an aqueous menstruum, it can be administered to women who are sensitive to the oils commonly used in
other estrone products. You may obtain Estrone Aqueous
Suspension through your pharmacy in 1-cc. ampoules
containing 2.0 mg. of pure crystalline estrone.
ABBOTT LABORATORIES, NORTH CHICAGO, ILL.

1. Freed, S. C., and Greenhill, J. P. (1941), J. Clin. Endocrinol., 1:983, December.

1946

Estrone Aqueous Suspension, 2.

at least not at individualized, low doses for short-term relief. Northrup suggests that bioidentical hormones, as well as dietary supplementation, are two viable options for women who are understandably leery of not only the symptoms of menopause, but of the conventional "cure" itself.

For the record, I will miss my period. I usually get it on the seventh of every month, and have so since I was ten. I like feeling in the cycle of my body.

— *Harriet F.* (47)

For those of us lucky enough to get old, menopause is a lot like menarche: it's definitely something we will all experience, sooner or later. And like a ten-year-old girl reading *Are You There God? It's Me, Margaret* for the first time, we may well feel frightened about the whole thing, or curious, or resigned, or oddly at peace with it. Mostly, we probably all have questions: When will it start? What will it feel like? How long will it last? And how will I feel when I'm not menstruating anymore?

HORMONAL BINGO

WRINKLES	FALLEN ARCHES	HIGH FIBER DIET	WATER RETENTION	GRAY HAIR
LIPOSUCTION	HORMONAL MOUSTACHE	DENTURE CREAM	VARICOSE VEINS	DOUBLE CHIN
MEMORY LOSS	ESTROGEN		CELLULITE	SHORT FUSE
HOT FLASH	FAD DIETS	BLOATING	LIVER SPOTS	GIRDLE
THIGH CREAM	MOOD SWINGS	PMS	SWOLLEN ANKLES	ERRATIC MOOD SWINGS

And yet, wouldn't it be wonderful never having to worry about birth control ever again? Or about getting pregnant? No more bleeding . . . couldn't that be liberating? And what about not having to buy another pad or tampon? To not have to worry about leaks, cramps, and hot flashes? To never need to run to the drugstore in a panic for either a box of tampons or a pregnancy test?

At least menopause, as a subject, is no longer hidden in some drawer along with the old underwear. Perimenopausal, menopausal, and postmenopausal women wanting information constitute a huge market, and businesses are looking to cash in. Just go online to a good search engine and type in "menopause"—you'll practically crash your computer from all the hits. It's possible to buy wisdom journals and T-shirts that say things like HELP . . . WHO TURNED UP THE HEAT?! and RED HOT MAMA, find special diet, exercise, and yoga programs, learn how to reinvent one's sex life. There's even a Chicken Soup book for the menopausal soul. One can determine one's "menopause type," learn tricks to combat cognitive losses, research Chinese medicine therapies—even get tips on surviving male menopause, as if one's own weren't enough. One can amuse oneself with *Menopop* (a pop-up and activity book), or buy menopause-specific sleepwear, pillowcases designed to quickly wick sweat away, or a subliminal programming CD designed to alleviate menopausal symptoms. One can browse skin-care products developed especially for menopausal (we're not sure if that's much better than "aging") skin and find lubricants to help make sex fun again. One can even order tickets to see *Menopause—The Musical*, which has been playing around the country since 2001. Or if not, one can buy the CD and songbook.

> *I love passing the feminine hygiene product aisle and knowing that's one less thing I need to buy. I feel as though I've paid my dues and I made it through. I wouldn't go back if you paid me. I love not getting my period.*
> —*Stacey S.* (53)

While some of the above may sound silly or even exploitative, we're heartened by the fact that at least women are talking about menopause and perhaps learning to accept it as an inevitable part of life. Hey, we're not suggesting it's supposed to be a day at Six Flags for everyone . . . but at least thanks to the ongoing dialogue, information, and even humor, menopause is no longer seen as the catastrophic end of a woman's life. Instead, it's becoming what it should have been all along: just another change.

> *I think I will be as excited as I was the first time I got my period—very happy and very proud to have reached this milestone.*
> —*Julia B.* (47)

I'M STILL HOT IT JUST COMES IN FLASHES NOW

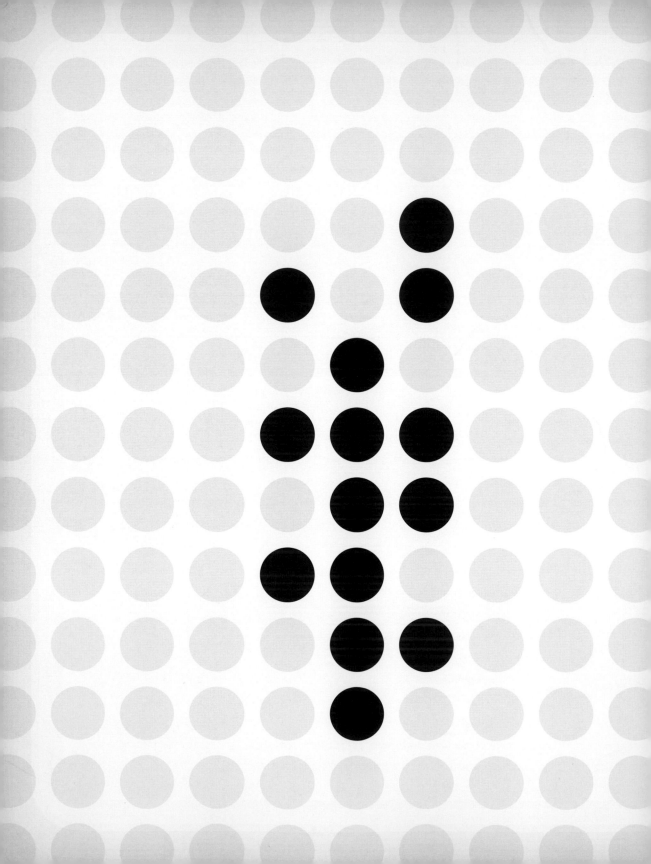

Chapter 14

OUTSIDE THE BOX

IN 1980, COMMERCIAL FEMCARE WAS SWEPT UP in a nationwide scandal. Thirty-eight girls and women had died of Toxic Shock Syndrome (TSS), a rare blood infection brought on by new-and-improved, superabsorbency tampons like Procter & Gamble's Rely (whose ad line, creepily enough, was "It even absorbs the worry").

Since then, all tampon manufacturers have phased out the most harmful ingredients. They also implemented a standardized absorbency rate and started plastering their packaging with dire warnings about TSS symptoms (sudden fever, vomiting, diarrhea, aches). Yet despite these precautions, there are still cases of TSS floating around. The official Web site of Stayfree, not what you'd call a hotbed of menstrual activism, says that one to seventeen of every 100,000 menstruating females will contract TSS *every year* (although these days, few cases are fatal).

As if that weren't enough to lose Jane Menstruator sleep, there's also the possible presence of dioxin in tampons. Dioxin isn't a single thing, but a family of chemical compounds, a very mean and evil family that are highly carcinogenic and toxic. Dioxins build up in animal tissue, where they just stay on and on and on, like extremely undesirable house guests.

Repeated tests have revealed only trace amounts of dioxin in tampons, well below the threshold that causes cancer. And yet talking about "a really small amount of dioxins" may be akin to calling someone "a little pregnant" or "kind of dead." After all, the stuff *does* build up. What's more, even though such low levels may not cause cancer, they might be linked to other problems, like endometriosis. None of this has been proven definitively, but it still gives one serious pause.

With the depressing realization that conventional, commercially available products can actually carry a drawback or two, including environmental ones (femcare products and packaging are a major contributor to landfills worldwide), women are understandably more open to exploring other options when it comes to dealing with menstrual flow, cramps, PMS, perimenopause, and postmenopause. And while we would never discount commercial products outright since far too many women (including us) rely on them, isn't it nice to have intriguing and often effective choices?

MYTH DEBUNKER

Worried about asbestos in your tampon? According to this widely spread online rumor, the major tampon companies have been sneaking the deadly material into their products just to make us bleed more. Dating back to the late 1970s, the asbestos-in-tampons rumor is emphatically just that, an urban myth along the lines of the camper who gets bitten by an insect and later has newly hatched baby spiders pouring out of his cheek. While tampons do contain other potentially troublesome ingredients like bleach, surfectants, waxes, alcohols, acids, and hydrocarbons, rest assured asbestos isn't one of them.

WACKIEST FEMCARE PRODUCTS

- A hormone replacement therapy album

- Rubber sanitary aprons

- A menopause pop-up book

- Baby wipes repackaged for women

- Hot flash pillowcases

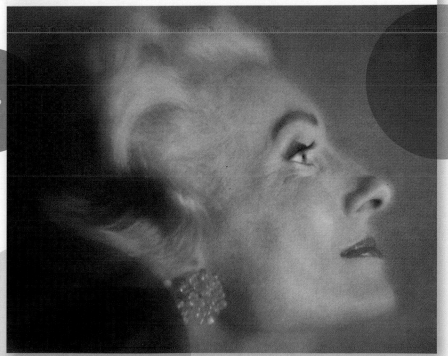

Current Concepts of Estrogen Replacement Therapy

How does the modern practitioner respond to the challenge of the menopause?

1966

Hormone therapy album   MCI

Take, for instance, the menstrual cup. First introduced, albeit not very successfully, in the 1930s, the menstrual cup is now beloved by many women who can't imagine a world without it. One can opt for the disposable kind, which is used once and then thrown away. Far more popular, however, is the reusable cup, which, if cared for properly, can last for up to ten years. There are numerous brands currently available online and in drugstores, including the Diva Cup, the Keeper, the Moon Cup, and Lunette.

Think about it . . . at roughly thirty bucks a pop, menstrual cups can be quite the bargain! And considering that the average woman will throw away 250 to 300 pounds of pads, plugs, and applicators in her lifetime, one would also save oneself significant guilt about dumping all that waste into our already-stressed environment. A menstrual cup can hold far more than any tampon, up to a full fluid ounce, making it a great option for heavy bleeders. It can be safely left in place

The menstrual cup is now beloved by many women who can't imagine a world without it.

for twelve hours, has never once been linked to TSS, is incapable of irritating or drying out the vagina, and what's more, it never leaks!

"So how does it work?" you may be grudgingly wondering. And just as important, what's the catch?

Made of silicone or rubber, a menstrual cup looks vaguely like a small, flexible Liberty Bell, minus the clapper and the crack. One folds the cup in half and inserts it (if one has ever used a diaphragm, one will immediately know what this entails); once inside, it pops open, creating an effective vacuum seal that keeps any blood from leaking out. To get it out, one must break the seal with one's finger and carefully yank it out, which can be a tad tricky and may on one's first attempt send bloody goo flying in all directions. Then one dumps out the contents, rinses it thoroughly, and reinserts.

Ta-da!

The catch isn't a catch to those who use it regularly and swear by its ease and comfort; and yet there are many of you out there (you know who you are) who are already shaking your heads in an emphatic "no." All that touching, all that inserting! Besides, who wants to handle her own blood that intimately? What's more, for heavy bleeders in the workplace, the thought of possibly having to wash one's menstrual cup out in a communal sink is about as appealing as seeing someone floss her teeth on the subway. Perhaps this is why the menstrual cup has never gone mainstream in America and continues to wait patiently in the wings for its big launch.

Another product that didn't quite make it was the Padette. A so-called interlabial pad, it was launched in 1995, and from the early reviews, one would have thought the company had found a cure for cancer. The Padette was a strange mutant, part pad, part tampon, and not quite either. Specifically, it was a small, oval pad, a mere three inches in length, that was designed to be held in place comfortably by one's labia. When a woman was standing or sitting, the labia would hold the pad in place; when she was on the toilet, the pad would fall out on its own, where it could be flushed away. Best used for short spells on light days, the Padette was beloved by the few who tried it, but then quickly disappeared. As of early 2008, it's currently being reintroduced as the Unique miniform.

Some women prefer sea sponges to soak up their flow. Sea sponges aren't plants, but literally sponge-like creatures—just about the lowest form of primitive animal life around—that grow in colonies on the ocean floor. Sea sponges work just like tampons, without applicators or strings for removal. To use, one merely squishes one up and inserts it into the vagina, where it expands as it soaks up blood. To remove, one pulls it out, rinses off

Above: Courtesy of Diva International, Inc.

the blood, and pops it back in. After air drying, it's ready for the next cycle.

As with the menstrual cup, reusability is a big plus— a sponge can last about six months or so—but some women find that they leak more than tampons. What's more, bacteria can build up, so one's sponge needs to be periodically soaked in vinegar and water or peroxide to be kept safe. And not to make one lose one's appetite or anything, but sponges, natural organisms that they are, have been found to contain sand, bacteria, grit, and other tiny, gnarly substances that one should definitely *not* be introducing into one's vagina.

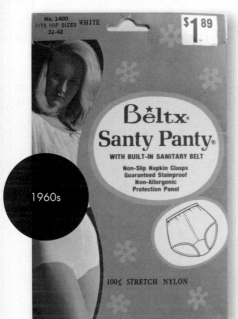

No. 1400
FITS HIP SIZES   WHITE
32-42

$1 89

Běltx.
Santy Panty.
WITH BUILT-IN SANITARY BELT

Non-Slip Napkin Clasps
Guaranteed Stainproof
Non-Allergenic
Protection Panel

100% STRETCH NYLON

1960s

Back in the 1960s, before adhesive strips changed femcare forever, clever manufacturers came up with sanitary panties and "panty-kinis" (a bikini-bottom-inspired style marketed to teens) that held pads in place, rather than the traditional cumbersome, homely belts and pins. Today, some smaller companies have taken that idea one step further and sell all-in-one "period panties," made with extra padding sewn permanently into the crotch. Some, made specifically for lighter days, are advertised as being a substitute for panty liners or shields. And others are designed to hold extra layers of fabric, also reusable, in the crotch to catch one's flow. After use, all can be thrown in the laundry.

One can also buy reusable pads that have extra sewn-in layers to soak up blood. Reusable cloth pads are nothing new; after all, women throughout history used them, and in fact, millions still do around the world. The upside? Many women find reusable pads, generally made out of flannel or other soft cotton, to be supercozy and comfortable. They're available in a variety of fabrics and patterns—crafty women can even make their own, downloading free patterns from the Internet and firing up the Singer. Plus, cloth pads can be used for years and contribute zilch to landfills.

Ecologically speaking, that's terrific. The downside is that they take work. Using cloth pads for years and years means you have to wash them for years and years. Generally speaking, one first soaks them in cold water and then throws them in with the laundry. Frequently, they also need a good hand scrubbing first to get rid of those stubborn bloodstains. All together, this can mean a lot more effort than some women want to give . . . and unless one already does a lot of laundry regularly, it can also lead to increased amounts of detergent being dumped into the waterways. As a result, some women find the best compromise is to use cloth pads (or other alternate femcare) only part of the time: at night, or on light days.

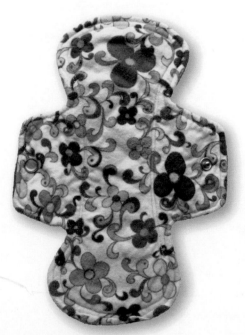

In the spirit of book research and eco-conservation, I delved into the world of reusable pads. There is quite a selection out there, and after much debating, vintage robots and groovy psychedelic flowers were my patterns of choice. They were fun to play with (snap on, snap off, snap on, snap off), and my kids found a variety of uses other than their intended purposes. Unfortunately, August was test month, and when it was ninety-plus degrees, all that flannel between my legs felt remarkably like wearing a hot and sweaty diaper. The total turn-off, though, was after using one. Seeing blood seeping into that pale blue background, covering those robots' little bodies, was too reminiscent of a lifetime of leaks—I had flashbacks of frantically trying to get rid of stains from my white carpenter pants before they set and ruined them forever. But no matter how much Ivory soap, scrubbing, and soaking, that faint brownish stain (then, and now) never went away. Perhaps it's been too many years of bleached-white, hygienically sealed, disposable pads. Even though I theoretically wanted to cut down on consumption and not contribute as much nonbiodegradable material to landfills, in the end, I'm sticking with Always. With wings.

—Elissa S. (43)

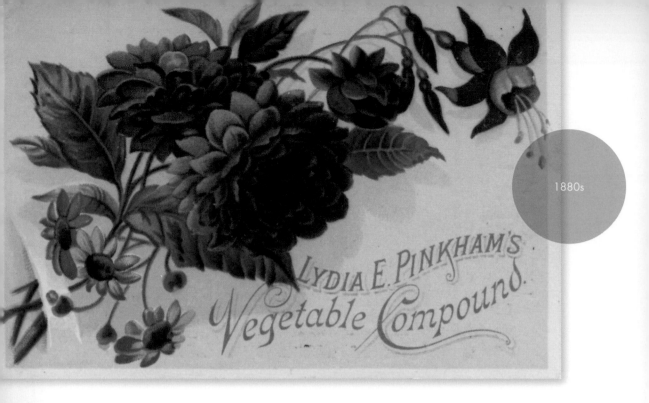

1880s

There are also alternative ways to deal with cramps and other unpleasant symptoms. Funnily enough, many of the out-there therapies currently in vogue are in fact nothing new, not by a long shot. For instance, herbal remedies for menstrual discomfort have not only been around for thousands of years, they were what all those midwives and village healers used to sling around in their bulging granny sacks. Eons before some guy in a suit came up with the name "Midol," these women were already pulling out the heavy herbal artillery to treat bloating, cramps, irregular periods, heavy bleeding, headaches, and skin problems, as well as to increase fertility, end pregnancies, and ease symptoms of menopause.

Black cohosh, for example, is a powerful plant that was used for years by Native Americans. A natural antispasmodic, anti-inflammatory, and natural sedative, it was practically made to fight menstrual discomfort, PMS, and the pain of childbirth. And according to the Mayo Clinic, it's also an effective treatment for numerous menopause symptoms, such as hot flashes, vaginal dryness, heart palpitations, and emotional swings.

Dong quai is a Chinese herb that's been effectively used for thousands of years. Best known as a muscle relaxant, it also tones and strengthens the uterus by causing it to contract before relaxing. A strong uterus is apparently a happy uterus; and a happy uterus means fewer menstrual cramps for the lucky female. Dong quai also appears to balance hormonal levels and helps regulate menstrual cycles that are out of whack.

Red raspberry leaf is another age-old star of the herbal hit parade and is said to promote a woman's health, not unlike dong quai, by strengthening her uterine walls. It's similarly recommended for relieving cramps and regulating periods. It's also suggested for use during pregnancy as it can ease nausea, help women relax during labor and delivery, and also get cycles back on track after birth.

Motherwort, ginseng, licorice, skullcap, ginger, dandelion, nettle, milk thistle, and pennyroyal . . . all of these are not only currently recommended to nonpregnant women for uterine health, symptom relief, and menstrual regularity, but were also routinely featured in certain patent medicines or nostrums, those mysterious and suspicious-looking elixirs and potions from the nineteenth century. In those heady days before federal regulations took all the fun out of healing, medicine makers didn't have to reveal what ingredients they used for their frequently demented claims; sure enough, some of the more dubious nostrums were eventually found to contain copious amounts of opium, cocaine, turpentine, camphor, and even radioactive materials. Yikes! Nevertheless, there were a few brands like Lydia Pinkham's Vegetable Compound, based on already-existing herbal remedies, that were much more benign and even pretty effective.

One popular patent medicine in the 1880s was manufactured by what would soon become one of the first pharmaceutical giants, Parke, Davis & Co. Called Chi-Ches-Ters, the tiny pill featured the you-catch-our-drift tagline "Chi-Ches-Ters turn 'problem' days into party days." Chi-Ches-Ters, which was on the market until the mid-1950s, contained such ingredients as cotton root bark, hellebore, iron sulfate, and aloe; chances are it originally contained cocaine, as well, but that was before they got all the kinks out. Cotton root bark, a common folk remedy among African slaves, is still used to help regulate menstrual flow. Similarly, cotton root bark and hellebore have also traditionally been used for menstrual disorders, iron sulfate is used to treat anemia, and aloe is a laxative. Altogether not the worst combination for dealing with some of the more annoying symptoms of menstruation!

Manufacturers now market a wide variety of menstrual and reproductive tonics and remedies, featuring several beneficial herbs all rolled into one package. You can even find premenstrual, pregnancy, hormonal-balancing, nursing, or female-toner tea/herbal combos in a cup. But before hotfooting it to one's local health food store, we suggest one spend some time reading, researching . . . and asking plenty of questions. Bestselling authors like Dr. Andrew Weil (*Women's Health: Ask Dr. Weil*), Dr. Christiane Northrup (*Women's Bodies, Women's Wisdom: Creating Physical and Emotional Health and Healing*), and Gary Null (*For Women Only: Your Guide to Health Empowerment*) suggest alternative therapies for all stages of female life, and theirs are just a few reputable voices of dozens, if not hundreds, out there.

There's encouraging word about vitamins and minerals, as well. *The American Journal of Obstetrics & Gynecology* notes that calcium and manganese, when taken together, significantly reduce mood swings, loss of concentration, and cramps during menstruation; they also reduce water retention during the premenstrual time. Vitamin E is said to regulate hormone levels and has been shown to significantly relieve breast tenderness and soreness. B-6 is a natural diuretic, which, trust us, comes in handy when menstrual bloat has turned one into an uncanny ringer for the Michelin Man.

And speaking of bloat, don't forget that something as simple as diet itself can make a huge difference. Cutting down on salt before your period can help you avoid all that unholy swelling. It's also known that constipation, not surprisingly, can make bad cramps even worse . . . so add that to the list of reasons one should consider adopting that high-fiber diet, washed down with plenty of water. Those who have discovered juicing also recommend a combination of apple, celery, and fennel juices to relieve menstrual cramps. Pineapple juice is said to relax muscles and help with cramps, as well.

Depending on how one feels about needles, some women swear by acupuncture as an effective way to relieve menstrual symptoms. For those of us more faint of heart, there's also acupressure and/or reflexology. Assuming one can commandeer the bathroom for an uninterrupted hour, one can also try hydrotherapy in the comfort of one's own home, soaking peacefully in a warm tub. Alternatively, cramps can often be relieved with hot

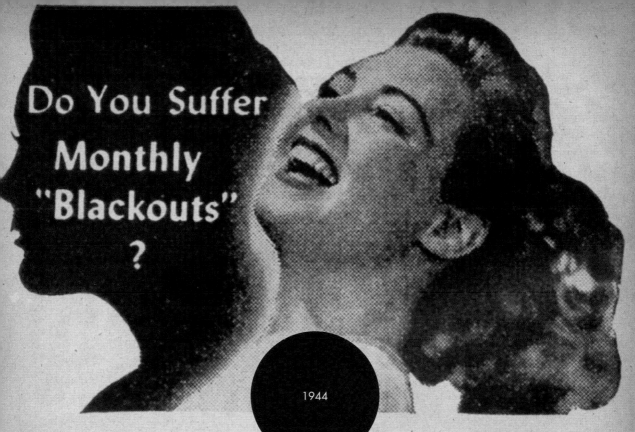

Do You Suffer Monthly "Blackouts"?

1944

Do functional periodic [pains] upset you? Try the preparation that's specially compounded for functional distress—the *new* Chi-Ches-Ters Pills. They've worked wonders for thousands of women. They should help you. For they do more than merely deaden pain. One of their ingredients tends to aid in relaxing the cramping and tension that causes distress. The added iron factor they contain is intended to help build up your blood, too. Ask your druggist today for a 50¢ box of the *new* Chi-Ches-Ters Pills. Then try them, as directed, for next month's "difficult days".

CHI-CHES-TERS PILLS

For relief from "periodic functional distress"

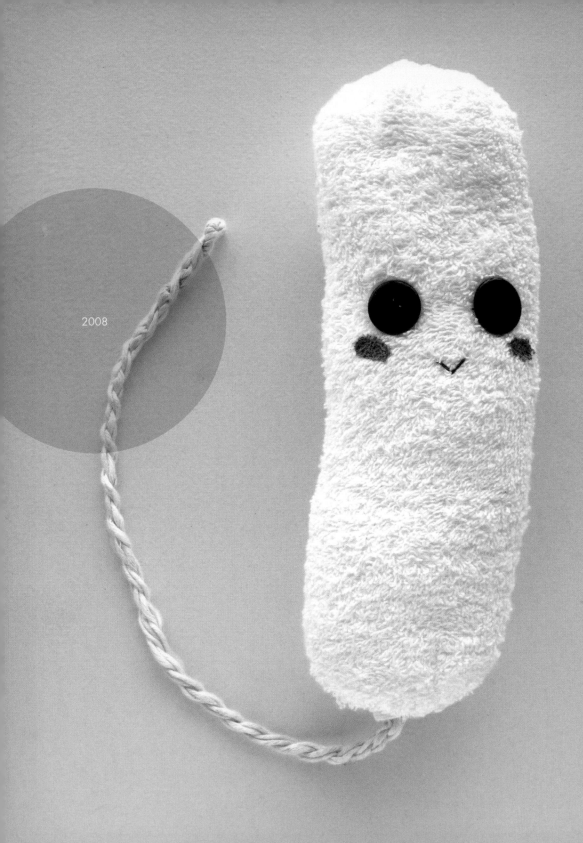

2008

water bottles or, funnily enough, even Ice packs. Massage, especially when focused on the pelvic region and lower back, works for many; we ourselves are especially fond of this treatment, even when we don't have cramps or aren't menstruating. In addition, there are numerous homeopathic and ayurvedic remedies one can try.

We hate to be the ones to add yet another reason why one should get off that couch, especially if one is feeling kind of tired and crampy, but the fact remains that exercise is one of the best ways around to deal with menstrual discomfort. We're not necessarily suggesting springing out the door and into a marathon (although Uta Pippig was visibly bleeding when she won her third consecutive Boston Marathon in 1996). Yet yoga, biking, swimming, dancing, hiking, and rock climbing all release endorphins, the naturally occurring "happy drug" in our brains, which can stop cramps cold. What's more, increased circulation and blood oxygen levels can help with pelvic discomfort. The same can be said of indoor sports. Menstrual sex may not be to everyone's liking, but the fact remains that orgasms are an effective, all-natural cramp reliever. Plus, they're free!

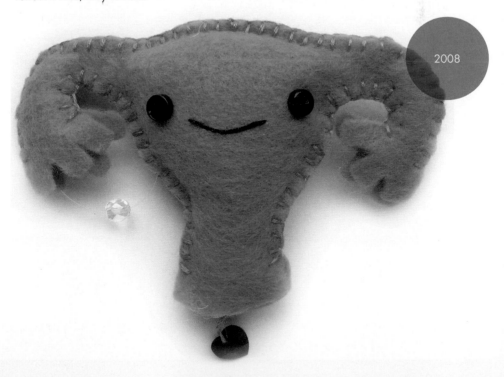

2008

Hands down, however, our favorite loopy therapy available online is special underwear outfitted with various magnets. According to the manufacturer, magnetic therapy reduces menstrual pain and PMS symptoms, although we have yet to be convinced. Nevertheless, we enjoy the image of coming home from work covered with loose paper clips and staples or, better yet, trying to talk one's way through airport security.

Speaking of alternative, there are also interesting things you can do with, believe it or not, your menstrual blood. Did you know one's flow can be used to fertilize plants? In *Her Blood Is Gold*, Lara Owen says she routinely soaks her used cloth pads in a covered bucket of cold water and then at the end of the week uses it in her garden. She also recommends bleeding on the ground from time to time, both to reconnect with and fertilize the earth. Rather than view her flow as waste, she instead reinterprets it as a powerful, nurturing substance. Her rationale is that when a woman is pregnant, all that extra blood and rich tissue goes to protecting a growing fetus. So why not put it to good use instead of flushing it down the toilet?

The underlying notion—that there's something potentially useful about our flow—is not as loopy as it may first sound. In fact, it's currently being explored by researchers who have recently discovered that menstrual blood contains certain types of stem cells. Potentially, endometrial stem cells could be used to combat a host of diseases and would be arguably less controversial, to some, than those obtained from human embryos.

The importance of menstrual flow was taken to new heights in 1993's *Blood, Bread, and Roses: How Menstruation Changed the World*. In her book, author Judy Grahn reinterprets all of history and cultural development from the standpoint that just about everything—from the invention of eating utensils, shoes, and furniture, to the notion of time, the origins of science, and human consciousness itself—somehow arose in direct response to menstruation. While one might certainly find fault with Grahn's menstrucentric thesis (we ourselves are a tad skeptical, considering that bleeding women have basically been treated like dog poop throughout history), it's nevertheless a thoughtful and creative attempt to recognize and honor women and their cycles.

There is, in fact, an underground movement of sorts to celebrate the female reproductive cycle and to bring it into the mainstream. Grassroots organizations, alternative

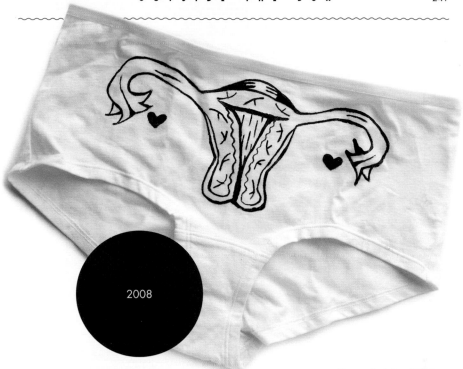

2008

Hearts and Lady Parts © Erin Seery

workshops, Web sites, books, and zines have sprung up over the last twenty years, trying to creatively and spiritually conquer the shame that's been ingrained in us for thousands of years.

Heal the Womb workshops, thrown by the Magick School in London, include such activities as massaging and positioning your own womb, as well as making "heal the womb" charm bags and your own personal goddess menses. One can pick up sacral chakra dancing, learn about herbs and crystals for feminine energy, or even paint one's belly to celebrate one's goddess belly.

Red Moon Rites of Passage endeavors "to empower your journey of making peace with your menstrual cycle, inspire you to welcome a girl into womanhood with ease and authenticity, and guide you to deeply appreciate your being a woman." Their goal is to help women recover from years of anger, frustration, embarrassment, and nonacceptance of their menstrual cycles, so they can then support girls they know from a positive and accepting place. They've started a training program for women to develop a closer spiritual relationship with their cycles and to eventually lead their own "coming of age" and "menstrual empowerment" ceremonies.

While Web sites tend to be launched and then wither away like dandelions in springtime, the trend of menstrucentric sites doesn't seem to be fading. Right now at womanwisdom.com, one can buy a home-study course with topics including the shamanic power of menstruation, sacred geometry, the wisdom and madness of menstrual taboos, the eroticism of blood mysteries, and menopause as a second puberty. One can also buy a guided meditation CD, goddess gowns in various colors, ceremonial crowns, even a menarche kit containing a jewelry-making project, workbooks, and a DVD.

2008

I was ten years old. I was on vacation, without my parents, with my cousins in Oklahoma. We were vacationing on a lake—swimming/waterskiing, etc. Even though I knew quite well what a period was and it was normal and nothing to be frightened of, I was horrified! I didn't tell my aunt or anyone else and I kept making excuses why I wouldn't go in the water. I kept stuffing toilet paper in my underwear. Finally, my aunt found out and of course helped me and called my mom, who I also spoke to. I felt much better once everyone knew and helped me. When I got home, my mom bought me a beautiful turquoise and silver ring to commemorate the occasion. I love that ring!

—Sarah B. (44)

When it comes to menarche, we ourselves have not actually participated in but have heard tales of red parties—where the food is red, the presents are red, and everyone wears red—all to celebrate a girl's first period. Knowing the girls in our lives, we think this could be seen as either a wonderful, empowering event that will be treasured forever or "the most humiliating thing that ever happened to me." Yet isn't at least the attempt to inject some celebration into a major life event preferable to the usual cultural hazing ceremony of fear, shame, and ignorance?

And how much more celebration can one imagine than *105 Ways to Celebrate Menstruation*? In her book, herbalist Kami McBride encourages women to acknowledge and appreciate monthly changes and cycles, instead of sweeping them perfunctorily under the rug while pretending they're not happening.

Above: Pink Uterus © Claire Elizabeth Platt

In 2007, the environmentally friendly company Seventh Generation launched tampontification.com, on which people could "virtually" donate femcare supplies to homeless shelters: each click would send a package of chlorine-free pads and tampons to women in need. The link went viral, as thousands of women forwarded it to their friends, families, and coworkers (we know we did); overwhelmed by the extraordinary response, Seventh Generation had to suspend the program until further notice.

> *Femcare has been so long monopolized by manufacturing, medicine, advertising, and religion that any fresh, individual voices seem like cool water in a blazing desert.*

There are so many menstrual-related Web sites, products, workshops, and support groups online, it's hard to keep track of them all. One can buy menstrual art that's been painted with actual blood. One can read about cultural rituals in which menstrual blood is used to attract men or keep them faithful. One can be even fringier and check out Web sites for those interested in "vampire play," where it's suggested that imbibing menstrual blood is an easy and painless way to quench one's thirst. One can read about how the act of performing oral sex on a menstruating woman is called getting one's "red wings." And for those interested in even kinkier stuff, one can check out eroticred.com, which features "homemade sexy, natural, & fun menstruation porn created by a variety of hot models of all shapes and styles on their periods!" There's even the Menstrual Avenger, an online cartoon heroine who can be found fighting evil with nothing more than a tampon lasso, a flying pad, and (when all else fails) her powerful, fire-hydrant-esque flow.

We couldn't write a book about menstruation without mentioning the Museum of Menstruation, an online treasure trove of menstrual history, information, and artifacts created and run by Harry Finley. For four years, the museum was housed in the basement of his suburban Washington, D.C., house (one of us recalls walking down his steep, slightly spooky basement steps and finding female mannequin torsos, decked out in historical menstrual gear, disconcertingly hanging from the ceiling), but now it exists strictly in cyberspace, at mum.org.

Finley is the go-to guy for all kinds of menstrual facts, opinions, and research. He's been quoted in *The New York Times*, featured on *The Daily Show*, and written up in *Bust* magazine. He was also the subject of a Sylvia comic strip, interviewed by Howard Stern, and consulted as an underwear expert (his site also covers the evolution of underwear) when Britney Spears flashed the paparazzi.

Mum.org is totally unique and absolutely riveting. One could spend days (and trust us, we have) exploring its strangely nonlinear layout, bouncing from patent medicine ingredients to visitors' quotes, vintage ads, art created with menstrual blood, then over to Harry's personal collection of cat photos. It's an extraordinary, albeit highly idiosyncratic and subjective, forum. And okay, if one was maybe expecting the Smithsonian, one can certainly pick at the Museum of Menstruation for all kinds of reasons (that it's run by a guy, that it's disorganized, that it's so utterly opinionated, that it's even called "mum" in the first place), but that's missing the point. Harry Finley's collection is really the only extensive repository of a pretty remarkable aspect of women's history . . . and that's worth a shout-out, no?

Another male voice in the menstrual world is Vinnie, as in *Vinnie's Giant Roller Coaster Period Chart & Journal Sticker Book*. The book contains charts and stickers to help keep track of first and last days, when friends are menstruating, and mood and body changes. Fans can also pick up *Vinnie's Cramp-Kicking Remedies* and Vinnie's Tampon Case.

So what do we make of men horning in on our body processes and, in Vinnie's case, turning a handy buck? Our feeling is, they've already been doing that for centuries, and at least Harry Finley and Vinnie are, relatively anyway, forces of good as opposed to evil. What's more intriguing to us is the overriding idea that femcare has been so long monopolized by the same monstrous juggernaut of manufacturing, medicine, advertising, and religion that any fresh, individual voices seem like cool water in a blazing desert.

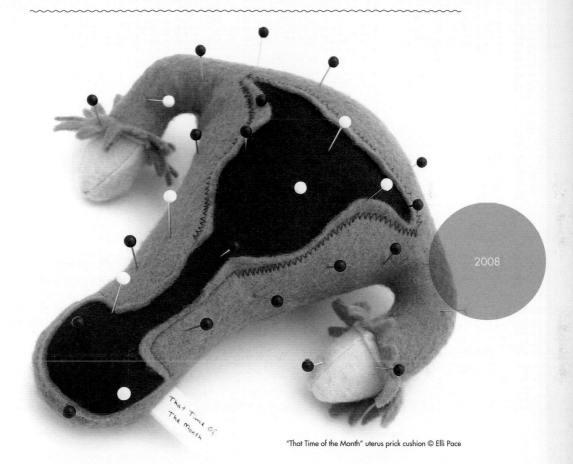

"That Time of the Month" uterus prick cushion © Elli Pace

Think about the young women who created Tampaction, a campaign of the Student Environmental Action Committee. Their goal? "To destroy patriarchal taboos, end environmental degradation caused by disposable tampons and pads, and promote vaginal and menstrual health." They spread their message in strictly grassroots terms, by encouraging fellow students to educate themselves about the products they're using and then share that information about alternatives on their campuses.

Blood Sisters (bloodsisters.org) promotes menstrual activism by encouraging women to bring product concerns to the attention of both femcare manufacturers and government officials. They also encourage experimentation with alternative products. They've hosted "Be Rad, Make a Pad," "Ax Tampax," and "D.I.Y. Gyno" workshops, produced the zine *Red Alert*, and continue to provide downloadable make-your-own-reusable-pad instructions on their Web site.

While menstruation is almost never mentioned in mainstream culture, it's amazing to see what's going on below the radar. There are zines, Web sites, YouTube videos, MySpace pages, and performance art pieces, all exploring the physical, psychological, and emotional aspects of menstruation with intelligence, activism, outrage, sensitivity, anger, and humor.

So what do we make of all this?

Don't get us wrong . . . we're thrilled to see that conversations are actually happening and that the female cycle is experiencing a sort of renaissance and is even occasionally celebrated. But to be totally blunt, we also find ourselves vaguely depressed by the very fringe-iness of goddess bowls, womb-healing circles, goddess rituals, and other ultra-alternative stuff. Because ultimately we wonder: alternative to what?

It's depressing that feeling comfortable in our own bodies is still considered so damn freaky and that exploring viable options to corporate femcare immediately puts one smack in the middle of some cultish, feminist ghetto. Nevertheless, we're hopeful since we know that we can each make an actual difference in our own lives. The way to start is by questioning assumptions, asking questions, and seeking out more information. Knowledge, after all, is powerful stuff. Let it work its magic by filtering into the conversations we have, informing the decisions we make, influencing the products we buy, and, last, shaping the lessons we pass on to our friends, colleagues, sisters, daughters, and granddaughters.

There are millions of women out there—mainstream women, women like you, women like us—who get along with the uterus just fine, along with all its bleeding, symptoms both good and bad, hormones, pregnancy fears and dreams, menarche, menopause, and the whole menstrual time line of our lives. With our new knowledge, we can hopefully take back a process that's been fundamentally ours all along, an indisputable part of our lives that has been too long judged, ridiculed, and hidden away.

Just go with the flow.

Bibliography

BOOKS

Angell, Marcia. *The Truth About the Drug Companies: How They Deceive Us and What to Do About It*. New York: Random Trade Paperbacks, 2005.

Angier, Natalie. *Woman: An Intimate Geography*. New York: Anchor-Random, 2000.

Bettelheim, Bruno. *The Uses of Enchantment: The Meaning and Importance of Fairy Tales*. New York: Vintage-Random, 1977.

Blume, Judy. *Are You There God? It's Me, Margaret*. New York: Bantam, 1970.

Boston Women's Health Book Collective, The. *The New Our Bodies, Ourselves*. New York: Touchstone, 1984.

Buckley, Thomas, and Alma Gottlieb. *Blood Magic: The Anthropology of Menstruation*. Berkeley: University of California Press, 1988.

Chrisler, Joan C., ed. *From Menarche to Menopause: The Female Body in Feminist Therapy*. New York: Haworth, 2004.

Coutinho, Elsimar M., with Sheldon J. Segal. *Is Menstruation Obsolete?* New York: Oxford University Press, 1999.

Dalton, Katharina, *Once a Month: The Premenstrual Syndrome. What It Is and How to Free Yourself from Its Effects*. Pomona: Hunter, 1979.

Dalton, Katharina, and Wendy Holton. *Once a Month: Understanding and Treating PMS*. Alameda, CA: Hunter, 1999.

Delaney, Janice, Mary Jane Lupton, and Emily Toth. *The Curse: A Cultural History of Menstruation*. Urbana: University of Illinois Press, 1988.

Dixon, Edward H. *Woman and Her Diseases, From the Cradle to the Grave: Adapted Exclusively to Her Instruction in the Physiology of Her System and All the Diseases of Her Critical Periods*. Philadelphia: Potter, 1866.

Ehrenreich, Barbara, and Deirdre English. *For Her Own Good: 150 Years of the Experts' Advice to Women*. New York: Doubleday, 1978.

Elson, Jean. *Am I Still a Woman? Hysterectomy and Gender Identity*. Philadelphia: Temple University Press, 2004.

Friedan, Betty. *The Feminine Mystique*. New York: Dell, 1964.

Golub, Sharon. *Periods: From Menarche to Menopause*. Newbury Park, U.K.: Sage, 1992.

Grahn, Judy. *Blood, Bread, and Roses*. Boston: Beacon, 1993.

Grimm, Jacob, Wilhelm Grimm, and Maria Tatar, trans. and ed. *The Annotated Brothers Grimm*. New York: Norton, 2004.

Hood, Mary G., M.D. *For Girls and the Mothers of Girls: A Book for the Home and the School Concerning the Beginnings of Life*. Indianapolis: Bobbs-Merrill, 1914.

Houppert, Karen. *The Curse: Confronting the Last Unmentionable Taboo: Menstruation*. New York: Farrar, 1999.

Kissling, Elizabeth Arveda. *Capitalizing on the Curse: The Business of Menstruation*. Boulder, CO: Rienner, 2006.

Latimer, Caroline Wormeley. *Girl and Woman*. New York: Appleton, 1909.

Lee, Joseph M. *Digest of Hygiene: A Woman's Life*. Joliet, IL: Modern Film Distributors, 1957.

Lein, Allen. *The Cycling Female: Her Menstrual Rhythm*. San Francisco: Freeman, 1979.

Maines, Rachel P. *The Technology of Orgasm: "Hysteria," the Vibrator, and Women's Sexual Satisfaction*. Baltimore: Johns Hopkins University Press, 1999.

Maxwell, W. H. *A Female Physician to the Ladies of the United States: Being a Familiar and Practical Treatise on Matters of Utmost Importance Peculiar to Women. Adapted for Every Woman's Own Private Use*. Self-published. 1860.

McGee Williams, Mary, and Irene Kane. *On Becoming a Woman*. New York: Dell, 1959.

Micale, Mark S. *Approaching Hysteria: Disease and Its Interpretations*. Princeton: Princeton University Press, 1995.

Northrup, Christiane. *The Wisdom of Menopause: Creating Physical and Emotional Health During the Change*. New York: Bantam, 2006.

Novak, Emil. *Menstruation and Its Disorders*. New York: Appleton, 1921.

Owen, Lara. *Her Blood Is Gold*. London: Aquarian–Harper Collins, 1993.

Palmer, Rachel Lynn, and Sarah K. Greenberg. *Facts and Frauds in Woman's Hygiene: A Medical Guide Against Misleading Claims and Dangerous Products*. New York: Vanguard, 1936.

Pemberton, Lois. *The Stork Didn't Bring You*. New York: Lion Library, 1955.

Peril, Lynn. *Pink Think: Becoming a Woman in Many Uneasy Lessons*. New York: Norton, 2002.

Pinkola Estés, Clarissa. *Women Who Run with the Wolves: Myths and Stories of the Wild Woman Archetype*. New York: Ballantine, 1992.

Shannon, T. W. *Self Knowledge and Guide to Sex Instruction: Vital Facts of Life for All Ages.* Ohio: Mullikin, 1913.

Sperry, Lyman B. *Confidential Talks with Young Women.* New York: Revell, 1898.

Taylor, Dena. *Red Flower: Rethinking Menstruation.* Freedom, CA: Crossing, 1988.

Walker, Barbara G. *The Women's Encyclopedia of Myths and Secrets.* New York: HarperOne, 1983.

Weideger, Paula. *Menstruation & Menopause: The Physiology and Psychology, the Myth and the Reality.* New York: Knopf, 1976.

Wilson, Robert A. *Feminine Forever.* New York: Evans, 1966.

ARTICLES

"Drop in Breast Cancer May Reflect Decline in Hormone Use." *Harvard Women's Health Watch,* July 2007: 7.

"Hysterectomy Doesn't Harm—and May Help—Sexual Function." *Harvard Women's Health Watch*, August 2007: 3.

"Negotiating the 'Bio-identicals' Controversy." *Harvard Women's Health Watch*, April 2008: 1–2.

"Ovary Removal Linked to Risk for Dementia, Parkinsonism." *Harvard Women's Health Watch*, January 2009: 3.

Quinlan, Mary Lou. "Working Through Menopause." *More,* June 2007: 88–92.

Richardson, Martha K. "Is It Safe to Take a Pill That Eliminates Periods?" *Harvard Women's Health Watch*, September 2007: 8.

Surowiecki, James. "A Drug on the Market." *The New Yorker*, June 25, 2007: 40.

White, Mastin G., and Otis Gates. "Decisions of Courts in Cases Under Federal Food and Drugs Act, Washington D.C.—*Chicester Chemical Co. v. United States*, Ct. Appeals, D.C., 4/6/31." Government Printing Office, 1934.

BOOKLETS AND PAMPHLETS

"Accent on You," Tampax, 1960.

"Accent on You," Tampax, 1966.

"At What Age," Kotex, 1961.

"How Shall I Tell My Daughter," Personal Products Company (Modess), 1954.

"How Shall I Tell My Daughter," Personal Products Company (Modess), 1969.

"It's Time You Knew," Tampax, 1966.

"Nancy's First Day at Camp," Personal Products Company (Modess), 1941.

"One Girl to Another," Kotex, 1943.

"Periodic Cycle, The," Personal Products Company (Modess), 1940.

"Personal," Lysol, 1942.

"Personal Hygiene," Kotex, 1928.

"Strictly Feminine," Personal Products Company (Modess), 1969.

"That Day Is Here Again," Kotex, 1943.

"Very Personally Yours," Kotex, 1961.

"Women's Secrets," Certane, 1935.

"You're a Young Lady Now," Kotex, 1952.

ONLINE

Abramson, Zelda. "Losing Heart: The Estrogen Dilemma—Rethinking Health Research for
    Midlife Women." *Women's Health & Urban Life: An International and Interdisciplinary
    Journal*, May 2002, UTSC. http://www.utsc.utoronto.ca/~socsci/sever/journal/1.1/
    Abramson.html

Ad Access. Duke University Libraries Digital Collections, 2008. http://library.duke.edu/
    digitalcollections/adaccess/

Al-Shahada. "Islam and Menses—What You Need to Know." *Islam: The Modern Religion.*
    http://www.themodernreligion.com/women/w_menses.htm

Always. The Procter & Gamble Co., 2008. http://www.always.com/index.jsp

"Apocrypha, The." A True Church, May 1999. http://www.atruechurch.info/apocrypha.html

Apter, D., and R. Vihko. "Early Menarche, a Risk Factor for Breast Cancer, Indicates Early
    Onset of Ovulatory Cycles." *Journal of Clinical Endocrinology & Metabolism,* 1983.
    http://jcem.endojournals.org/cgi/content/abstract/57/1/82

Barrett, Jennifer. "Selling Sickness to the Well: A Newsweek Interview with Ray Moynihan."
    Newsweek, August 2, 2005. http://www.archivum.info/sci.med/2005/08/
    msg00152.html

Bearak, Barry. "Katmandu Journal; When Life as a Goddess Ends, Life as a Girl Begins." *New York Times*, December 12, 1998. http://query.nytimes.com/gst/fullpage.html?res= 9C03E0DE1F3AF931A25751C1A96E958260

Being Girl. The Procter & Gamble Co., 2008. http://beinggirl.com/en_US/home.jsp

Bettelheim, Matthew. "'That Time' In Evolutionary History." *Inkling*, January 31, 2007. http://www.inu.net/skeptic/origin.htm

"Black Cohosh: Healing Herb." The Cauldron. http://www.ecauldron.com/articles/ archives/2006/05/entry_36.php

Blood Sisters Project, The. http://bloodsisters.org/bloodsisters/

"Body: Getting Your Period." Girls Health. The National Women's Health Information Center, 2007. http://www.girlshealth.gov/body/period.htm

Bramshaw, Vikki. "The Moon in Religion and Mythology." The Witches' Voice, March 16, 2007. http://www.witchvox.com/va/dt_va.html?a=ukgb2&c=basics&id=11646

Brink, Susan. "Girl, You'll Be a Woman Sooner Than Expected." *Los Angeles Times*, January 21, 2008. http://www.cuttingthroughthematrix.com/articles/Girl_youll_be_a_woman_ sooner_than_expected.htm

Cablo, Louis W. "Human Sexuality and the Origin of Religion." Skeptics Corner. http:// www.inu.net/skeptic/origin.htm

Casselman, Bill. "Hysteria: The Just Death of a Medical Word." Bill Casselman's Canadian Word of the Day, August 2007. http://www.billcasselman.com/dictionary_of_medical_ derivations/fifteen_hysteria.htm

Cho, Margaret. "Why Must I Bleed Alone?" Margaret Cho blog. January 20, 2004. http://www.margaretcho.com/blog.htm?var1=http://www.margaretcho.com/blog/ whymustibleedalone.htm

Chrisler, Joan C., and Paula Caplan. "Strange case of Dr. Jekyll and Ms. Hyde: How PMS became a cultural phenomenon and a psychiatric disorder." *Annual Review of Sex Research*, 2002. http://findarticles.com/p/articles/mi_qa3778/is_200201/ ai_n9032351/pg_16

Chuppa-Cornell, Kim. "Filling a vacuum: women's health information in *Good Housekeeping*'s articles and advertisements, 1920–1965." *The Historian*, September 22, 2005. http://www.encyclopedia.com/doc/1G1-158156313.html

Citrinbaum, Joanna. "The question's absorbing: 'Are tampons little white lies?'" *Daily Collegian*, 2003. http://www.collegian.psu.edu/archive/2003/10/10-14-03tdc/ 10-14-03dscihealth-01.asp

Coco, Andrews. "Primary Dysmenorrhea." *American Family Physician*, August 1999. http://www.aafp.org/afp/990800ap/489.html

Cornforth, Tracee. "Menstruation 101." About.com, August 12, 2005. http://womenshealth.about.com/cs/menstruation/a/understandmenst.htm

Davoudi, Salamander. "Study casts doubt on anti-depressants." *Financial Times*, February 25, 2008. http://www.ft.com/cms/s/6fce3400-e3d5-11dc-8799-0000779fd2ac,Authorised=false.html?_i_location=http%3A%2F%2Fwww.ft.com%2Fcms%2Fs%2F0%2F6fce3400-e3d5-11dc-8799-0000779fd2ac.html%3Fnclickcheck%3D1&_i_referer=http%3A%2F%2Fwebmail.pas.earthlink.net%2Fwam%2Fmsg.jsp%3Fmsgid%3D14202%26folder%3DINBOX%26isSeen%3Dtrue%26x%3D946398944&nclick_check=1

DeLashmutt, Gary. "Romans 16:1-16—Paul's View of Women." Xenos Christian Fellowship, 2000. http://www.xenos.org/teachings/nt/romans/gary/rom16-1.htm

"DES: Questions and Answers." National Cancer Institute. http://www.cancer.gov/cancertopics/factsheet/Risk/DES

Donohue, Julie M., Marisa Cevasco, and Meredith B. Rosenthal. "A Decade of Direct-to-Consumer Advertising of Prescription Drugs." *New England Journal of Medicine*, August 16, 2007. http://content.nejm.org/cgi/content/full/357/7/673

"Drugs & Supplements." Mayo Clinic. http://www.mayoclinic.com/health/drug-information/DrugHerbIndex

"Early Years—Our History." Johnson & Johnson, 2008. http://www.jnj.com/our_company/history/history_section_1.htm

"Embryology: History of Embryology as a Science." Science Encyclopedia. http://science.jrank.org/pages/2452/Embryology.html

Erotic Red. http://www.eroticred.com/

"FAQs About Shorter Periods." Loestrin 24 Web site, 2008. http://www.loestrin24.com/faqs.php#shorter

"FDA Approves Lybrel, First Low Dose Combination Oral Contraceptive Offering Women the Opportunity to Be Period-Free over Time." Wyeth.com, May 22, 2007. http://www.wyeth.com/news?nav=display&navTo=/wyeth_html/home/news/pressreleases/2007/1179876879334.html

Ferguson, Susan J., and Carla Parry. "Rewriting menopause: Challenging the medical paradigm to reflect menopausal women's experiences." *Frontiers*, 1998. http://findarticles.com/p/articles/mi_qa3687/is_199801/ai_n8766412

Fewer Periods. Duramed Pharmaceuticals, Inc., 2006. http://www.fewerperiods.com

Finley, Harry. Museum of Menstruation, 2008. http://www.mum.org/; http://findarticles
.com/p/articles/mi_qa3687/is_199801/ai_n8766412/pg_1

Francoeur, Robert T., Ph.D. "Catholic Culture and Sexuality." Institutsserver WWW2. http://
www2.hu-berlin.de/sexology/GESUND/ARCHIV/catholic.htm

Fraser, Amy E. "Uterus: Sacred Sexuality and Feminine Symbolism." http://www.aefraser
.com/dtwwa/chapter9_uterus.htm

Frederick, Jenn. "The First Taboo: How Menstrual Taboos Reflect and Sustain Women's
Internalized Oppression." Cool Beans. http://home.comcast.net/~theennead/bean/
index.htm

Gallagher, Kathe, and Debby Golonka. "Endometrial Ablation." Web MD Web site,
February 22, 2006. http://women.webmd.com/endometrial-ablation-16200

Gauss, Julie. "Sacred Menstruation: Reclaiming the Power of Our Moontime." *Sentient Times*,
September 2004. http://www.sentienttimes.com/04/aug_sept_04/sacred.html

Grieve, M. "Cotton Root." *A Modern Herbal*, 1931. http://www.botanical.com/botanical/
mgmh/c/cotto109.html

Gunther, Kerry A. "Bears and Menstruating Women." Yellowstone, May 2002. http://www
.nps.gov/yell/naturescience/bears_women.htm

Have a Happy Period. The Procter & Gamble Co., 2008. http://www.always.com/happy/
home.jsp

Healy, Bernadine. "Estrogen Use: Less Confusion, More Clarity." *U.S. News & World Report*,
June 21, 2007. http://health.usnews.com/usnews/health/articles/070621/21healytip
.htm

Hippocrates. Trans. by Francis Adams. "Aphorisms." The Internet Classics Archive. http://
classics.mit.edu/index.html

"History of the Male and Female Genitalia." Stanford University. http://www.stanford.edu/
class/history13/earlysciencelab/body/femalebodypages/genitalia.html

Holmes, Hannah. "The Truth About Tampons." *Garbage*, Nov./Dec. 1990. http://www
.keeper-menstrual-cup.com/tampons_truth.html

"Hormone therapy: Introduction." Excerpted from *Essential Guide to Menopause*. American
Medical Association–Medem, 1998. http://www.medem.com/medlb/article_detaillb
.cfm?article_ID=ZZZACTPUCKC&sub_cat=0

Houppert, Karen. "Final Period." *New York Times*, July 17, 2007. http://www.nytimes
.com/2007/07/17/opinion/17houppert.html

Houppert, Karen. "Pulling the Plug on the Sanitary Protection Industry." *Village Voice*,

February 7, 1995. http://www.spotsite.org/village.html

"India Reassesses Menstrual Forms." BBC News, April 12, 2007. http://news.bbc.co.uk/2/hi/south_asia/6547909.stm

"Internal genital organs." Merck, 1995–2008. http://www.merck.com/mmhe/sec22/ch241/ch241c.html

Johnson, Philip S. "Sex and Spirituality." Jesus.com. http://www.jesus.com.au/html/page/sex_and_spirituality

Kaiser, Jocelyn. "FDA Oversight of Trials Found Lacking." *ScienceNOW Daily News*, September 28, 2007. http://sciencenow.sciencemag.org/cgi/content/full/2007/928/1

Katz, Leslie. "The Bloody Truth About Menstruation." *Oakland Tribune*, July 25, 2004. http://findarticles.com/p/articles/mi_qn4176/is_20040725/ai_n14579723/pg_1

Kerr, Martha. "Menstrual Blood Yields Stem Cells." *ABC Science*, March 15, 2006. http://www.abc.net.au/science/news/health/HealthRepublish_1590861.htm

Keshavarz, Homa, Susan D. Hillis, Burney A. Kieke, and Polly A. Marchbanks. "Hysterectomy Surveillance—United States, 1994–1999." Morbidity and Mortality Weekly Report, July 2, 2002. http://www.cdc.gov/mmwr/preview/mmwrhtml/ss5105a1.htm

Kinetz, Erika. "Is Hysteria Real? Brain Images Say Yes." *New York Times*, September 26, 2006. http://www.nytimes.com/2006/09/26/science/26hysteria.html?r=1&ex=1175140800&en=acd150e860c9cbc8&ei=5070&oref=slogin

King, Sue, Hemitra Crecraft, and Anne Strawbridge. Woman Wisdom. http://www.womanwisdom.com/

Know My Cycle. Wyeth Pharmaceuticals Inc., 2008. http://www.knowmycycle.com/

Kolata, Gina. "Books of the Times: On the Trail of Estrogen and a Mirage of Youth." Rev. of *The Greatest Experiment Ever Performed on Women: Exploding the Estrogen Myth* by Barbara Seaman. *New York Times*, July 5, 2003. http://query.nytimes.com/gst/fullpage.html?res=980CE6DF1F3AF936A35754C0A9659C8B63

"Lactational Amenorrhea Method." Planned Parenthood, November 1, 2006. http://www.plannedparenthood.org/issues-action/birth-control/bc-history-6547.htm

Lalloo, Sherneen. "Hindu Women and Sexuality." African Gender Institute, December 2000. http://web.uct.ac.za/org/agi/pubs/newsletters/vol7/sherne.htm

Lefkowitz, Mary R., and Maureen B. Fant. "Women's Life in Greece and Rome." The Stoa Consortium. http://www.stoa.org/diotima/anthology/wlgr/wlgr-medicine.shtml

Levine, Shari. "Where Are the Wise Women?" Girlzone. SheKnows.com, 2008. http://www.girlzone.com/insideout/Womanhood_io.html

Lord, M. G. "Litterbugs: A Study of Trash and How It Has Changed Our Culture." *New York Times*, September 19, 1999. http://query.nytimes.com/gst/fullpage.html?res=9D03E0DA143DF93AA2575AC0A96F958260&scp=8&sq=Litterbugs&st=nyt

MacLeod, Nadia. Menstruation.com.au, 2006. http://www.menstruation.com.au/periodpages/periodsmenu.html

Maloney, C. "Robin Danielson Act." 110th Congress, 2nd Session, January 29, 2008. http://thomas.loc.gov/cgi-bin/thomas

Mayo Clinic Staff. "Hot flashes: Minimize discomfort during menopause." Mayo Clinic, June 12, 2007. http://www.mayoclinic.com/health/hot-flashes/HO01409

McLaughlin, Daniel. "Poles Ban Sex and Beer on TV for Pope's Visit." *Guardian*, May 21, 2006. http://www.guardian.co.uk/world/2006/may/21/catholicism.religion

"Menarche, Menopause and Breast Cancer Risk: the Facts." Breakthrough Publications. http://www.breakthrough.org.uk/what_we_do/breakthrough_publications/menarche.html

Meng, Xiaolong, Thomas E. Ichim, Jie Zhong, Andrea Rogers, Zhenglian Yin, James Jackson, Hao Wang, Wie Ge, Vladimir Bogin, Kyle W. Chan, Bernard Thébaud, and Neil H. Riordan. "Endometrial regenerative cells: A novel stem cell population." *Journal of Translational Medicine*, November 15, 2007. http://www.translational-medicine.com/content/pdf/1479-5876-5-57.pdf

"Menopause: Myths and Medicine." Australian Broadcasting Company, 2000. http://www.abc.net.au/science/menopause/

"Menstrual Cycles: What Really Happens in Those 28 Days?!" Feminist Women's Health Center. http://www.fwhc.org/health/moon.htm

"Menstrual Problems." From *New Choices in Natural Healing*. Mother Nature. http://www.mothernature.com/Library/Bookshelf/Books/21/155.cfm

"Menstrual Products." Vagina Pagina. http://www.vaginapagina.com/index.php?title=Menstrual Products

"Menstruation and the Menstrual Cycle." Office on Women's Health, U.S. Department of Health and Human Services Web site, November 2002. http://www.4woman.gov/FAQ/menstru.htm

Mikkelson, Barbara. "Killer Sperm." Snopes.com, March 16, 2007. www.snopes.com/cokelore/sperm.asp

Mikkelson, Barbara and David P. "Asbestos in Tampons." Snopes.com, 2008. http://www
.snopes.com/medical/toxins/tampon.asp

Miller, Hannah. "Conversations with My Tampon: Do Women Really Need Uplifting
Messages from Their Menstrual Products?" *Salon*, September 1, 2004. http://dir.salon
.com/story/mwt/feature/2004/09/01/ditties/index1.html

Nelson, Emily, and Miriam Jordan. "Seeking New Markets For Tampons, Procter & Gamble
Tries 'Bonding Sessions' and School Slide Shows to Win Sales in Mexico." *Wall Street
Journal*, December 8, 2000. http://www.stayfreemagazine.org/public/wsj_tampons.html

Nicholas, Sadie. "The Women Who Use the Morning After Pill as Everyday Contraception."
The Daily Mail, October 3, 2007. http://www.dailymail.co.uk/pages/live/femail/
article.html?in_article_id=485303&in_page_id=1879

Nordqvist, Christian. "Contraceptive Pill May Lower a Woman's Cancer Risk." *Medical News
Today*, September 12, 2007. http://www.medicalnewstoday.com/articles/82217.php

o.b. The Procter & Gamble Co., 2008. http://www.obtampons.com/en/index.jsp

O'Grady, Kathleen, and Paula Wansbrough. "Celebrations." Canadian Women's Health
Network, 1997. http://www.cwhn.ca/resources/pub/Sweet_Secrets/celebrations.html

Olson, Eugénie. "Are Periods Passé? More Women Are Taking a Break from Menstruation."
Revolution Health, June 6, 2007. http://www.revolutionhealth.com/conditions/
reproductive-health/body/passe

"Ovaries or Not: Is Your Only Choice Between Ovarian Cancer and Surgical Menopause?"
A Survivor's Guide to Surgical Menopause, April 20, 2006. http://surmeno.blogspot
.com/2006/04/ovaries-or-not-is-your-only-choice.html

Paddock, Catharine. "Scientists Find Estrogen Protects Women's Brains." *Medical News
Today*, August 20, 2007. http://www.medicalnewstoday.com/articles/81132.php

Parker, William, M.D. "Problems with Your Periods." *A Gynecologist's Second Opinion.*
http://www.gynsecondopinion.com/period.htm

Parsons, Rhea. "Portrayal of PMS on Television Sitcoms, The." *MP: An Online Feminist
Journal*, December 2004. http://www.academinist.org/mp/mp_archive/archive/
december04/ampioa3.html

Peres, Judy. "Risks of hormone therapy decline over time, study finds." *Chicago Tribune*,
March 5, 2008. http://www.chicagotribune.com/news/local/chi_hormones_
webmar05,0,594646.story

"Pills to Keep Women Young." *Time*, April 1, 1966. http://www.time.com/time/magazine/
article/0,9171,840627-1,00.html

Playtex. Playtex Products Inc., 2007. http://www.playtexproductsinc.com/corppages/index.asp

"Postmenopausal hormones: Hormone therapy: What happened?" Harvard Medical School, 2008. http://www.health.harvard.edu/newsweek/Postmenopausal_hormones_ Hormone_therapy.htm

"Premenstrual Dysphoric Disorder (PMDD): What Is Premenstrual Dysphoric Disorder?" Medem—American Psychiatric Association, 2001. http://www.medem.com/MedLB/ article_detaillb.cfm?article_ID=ZZZF9KNGTRC&sub_cat=2003

"Premenstrual Syndrome." The American College of Obstetricians and Gynecologists, September 2003. http://www.medem.com/MedLB/article_detaillb.cfm?article_ ID=ZZZF9KNGTRC&sub_cat=2003

Project Aware, 2008. http://project-aware.org/index.shtml

The Red Spot. http://www.onewoman.com/redspot/index.html

"Reusable Menstrual Products," 2002–2007. http://www.labyrinth.net.au/~obsidian/ clothpads/index.htm

Robbins, John. "Menstrual Cycles and Sea Sponges." The Food Revolution. http://www .foodrevolution.org/askjohn/49.htm

Rocca, W. A., J. H. Bower, D. M. Maraganore, J. E. Ahlskog, B. R. Grossardt, M. de Andrade, and L. J. Melton III. "Increased Risk of Parkinsonism in Women Who Underwent Oophorectomy Before Menopause." *Neurology*, August 29, 2007. http:// www.neurology.org/cgi/content/abstract/01.wnl.0000280573.30975.6av1

Roderick, Kyle. "10 Myths Men Believe About Menopause." Third Age. http://www .thirdage.com/features/healthy/clueless/

Rola, Linda. "What causes early menopause and what causes menopause?" Safe Menopause Solutions. http://www.safemenopausesolutions.com/causesmenopause.html

Rubenstein, Sarah. "Wyeth Penalized $134.5 Million In Hormone-Replacement Verdict." *Wall Street Journal*, October 11, 2007. http://online.wsj.com/article/ SB119211221418156021.html?mod=googlenews_wsj

Ruth's Page: Endometriosis and Dioxin, 1997–2004. http://www.frontiernet.net/~ruthb/ Endometriosis.html

Sanghavi, Sarshak M. "Preschool Puberty, and a Search for the Causes." *New York Times*, October 17, 2006. http://www.nytimes.com/2006/10/17/science/17puberty .html?fta=y

Shorto, Russell. "Contra-Contraception." *New York Times Magazine*, May 7, 2006. http:// www.nytimes.com/2006/05/07/magazine/07contraception.html?ex=1304654400&

en=fd92772f01a5c709&ei=5088&partner=rssnyt&emc=rss

Singer, Michelle A. L. "Top Ten Things to Know About Menstruation." Lewis & Clark College Womyn's Center Web site, April 19, 2001. http://www.lclark.edu/~womynctr/Top10Things.html

Smith, Tovia. "Feminist Jews Revive Ritual Bath for Women." *NPR Weekend Edition*, July 9, 2006. http://www.npr.org/templates/story/story.php?storyId=5490415

Society for Menstrual Cycle Research Web site. http://menstruationresearch.org/

SPOT, the Tampon Health Website. http://www.spotsite.org/

Spriggs, William A. "Menstrual Odors, Dirty Diapers, and the Male Dominated Religious Quest for Purity: Giving Birth to Misogyny, Ethnic, and Racial Discriminations Originating in the Human Biological Emotion of Disgust." *Evolution's Voyage*, June 20, 2007. http://www.evoyage.com/BillsEssays/MenstrualOdors&Religion.htm

Stayfree Web site, McNeill-PPC, Inc., 2008. http://www.stayfree.com/index.jsp

Stevenson, Seth. "Can Tampons Be Cool? Playtex Gives Feminine Care a Sporty Makeover." *Slate*, January 15, 2007. http://www.slate.com/id/2157494/

Straight Dope Science Advisory Board. "Who Invented Tampons?" The Straight Dope, June 6, 2006. http://www.straightdope.com/mailbag/mtampons.html

Strovny, David. "Have Great Sex While She's Menstruating." Askmen.com. http://www.askmen.com/love/love_tip_60/61_love_tip.html

"Synthetic Hormone Used in Contraceptives and HRT Produces Negative Effects in Monkey Studies." *ScienceDaily*, June 8, 2004. http://www.sciencedaily.com/releases/2004/06/040608065645.htm

"Synthetic Hormone Used in Contraceptives, HRT Increases Aggression in Monkeys." *Synapse*, Summer 2004. http://www.cs.princeton.edu/~zkhan/popscience/summer2004.pdf

"Talmud Laws of Menstruation." Come and Hear: An Educational Forum for the Examination of Religious Truth and Religious Tolerance, 2003. http://www.come-and-hear.com/editor/america_3.html

"Tambrands Inc." Funding Universe. http://www.fundinguniverse.com/company-histories/Tambrands-Inc-Company-History.html

"Tampaction." Student Environmental Action Coalition Web site. http://www.seac.org/taxonomy/term/3

Tampax. The Procter & Gamble Co., 2008. http://tampax.com/

Tampax Upgrade U. The Procter & Gamble Co., 2008. http://tampax.com/upgradeu
.php?bg

"Tampons and Asbestos, Dioxin, & Toxic Shock Syndrome." FDA Web site, July 23, 1999.
http://www.fda.gov/cdrh/consumer/tamponsabs.html

Tampontification. Seventh Generation. http://www.tampontification.com/index.php

Taubes, Gary. "Do We Really Know What Makes Us Healthy?" *New York Times*, September
16, 2007. http://www.nytimes.com/2007/09/16/magazine/16epidemiology-t
.html?_r=1&oref=slogin

"Top 10 Intelligent Designs (or Creation Myths)." Live Science. http://www.livescience.com/
history/top10_intelligent_designs-1.html

Tumulty, Karen. "Jesus and the FDA." *Time*, October 14, 2002. http://www.time.com/time/
magazine/article/0,9171,1003443,00.html

"Urban Legends Reference Pages." Snopes.com. http://search.atomz.com/search/?sp-
q=menstruation&getit=Go&sp-a=00062d45-sp00000000&sp-advanced=1&sp-p=all&
sp-w-control=1&sp-w=alike&sp-date-range=-1&sp-x=any&sp-c=100&sp-m=1&sp-s=0

Uterus1. Body1, Inc., 2008. http://www.uterus1.com/

Veracity, Dani. "The Great Direct-to-Consumer Prescription Drug Advertising Con: How
Patients and Doctors Alike Are Easily Influenced to Demand Dangerous Drugs."
NaturalNews.com, July 31, 2005. http://www.naturalnews.com/010315.html

Vitale, Sidra. "Toxic Shock Syndrome." Web by Women, for Women, 1997. http://www
.io.com/~wwwomen/menstruation/tss.html

Voiland, Adam. "Illuminating Shark Exposure to Ecoestrogens." *Mote Magazine*, 2005.
http://www.mote.org/index.php?src=directory&srctype=display&view=magazine&i
d=704

"Vulvodynia." *Health Central Encyclopedia*, 2001–2008. http://www.healthcentral.com/
encyclopedia/408/274.html

Warkentin, Elyssa. "Selling Shame: Subversive advertising of menstrual products." *The
Manitoban*, November 7, 2001. http://themanitoban.com/2001-2002/1107/features
6.shtml

Weil, Andrew, M.D. "Herbs for Menopause Symptoms and Menopause Treatment." Dr. Weil
Web site. http://www.drweil.com/drw/u/ART00700/menopause-symptoms

West, Sharon K. "A Visit from Auntie." Suite 101, March 24, 2004. http://www.suite101
.com/article.cfm/history_bizarre_mysterious/107345

Will, Barbara. "The Nervous Origins of the American Western." *American Literature*, June

1998. http://www.jstor.org/pss/2902839

Williams, Monnica. Epigee Women's Health, 2008. http://www.epigee.org/

"Witches Every Month." *Time*, October 22, 1956. http://205.188.238.109/time/
    magazine/article/0,9171,824519,00.html

Witcombe, Christopher L.C.E. "Women in the Aegean: Minoan Snake Goddess." Dr.
    Christopher L.C.E. Witcombe, 2008. http://witcombe.sbc.edu/snakegoddess/
    snakecharmers.html

Women Priests: The Case for Ordaining Women in the Catholic Church. http://www
    .womenpriests.org/index.asp

Woolley, John T., and Gerhard Peters. "Calvin Coolidge: Address Before the American
    Association of Advertising Agencies, Washington, D.C." The American Presidency
    Project, 2008. http://www.presidency.ucsb.edu/ws/print.php?pid=412

Yeung, Dannii Y. L. "Psychosocial and Cultural Factors Influencing Expectations of Menarche:
    A Study on Chinese Premenarcheal Teenage Girls." *Journal of Adolescent Research—*
    Sage Publications, 2005. http://jar.sagepub.com/cgi/content/refs/20/1/118

Zajacz, Maria. "Dr. Swift's Cure for Hysteria." Explore Historic California. http://www
    .explorehistoricalif.com/hysteria.html

Acknowledgments

Endless thanks to Victoria Sanders, our agent, and Rose Hilliard, our editor, whose encouragement, enthusiasm, and exquisite professionalism made *Flow* a reality. Thanks to Paul Kepple, for his extraordinary design, and to Lisa Pompilio, for creating *Flow*'s stunning cover.

Many thanks to Trina Robbins, yet again, for sharing her amazing collection of vintage women's magazines with the world. We would also like to thank Ellie Young and Wanda Husick at decodog.com for finding the elusive ads that help tell the story so well; Laurie Henzel at *Bust* for opening her vintage magazine archive; Susan Carskadon at Diva International, Inc.; Dr. William Fleming at Unique Miniforms; Dr. Shelley Kolton; the informative staff at the New York City Public Library Picture Collection; and Mitch Evans of Ad*Access, at Duke University Libraries.

Much appreciation to the following artists for allowing us to include their work: Amanda Adams, Erin Seery, Kristen St. Thomas, Claire Elizabeth Platt, Elli Pace, and Bredette Dyer.

We'd also like to thank Jennifer Enderlin, John Murphy for "getting it" with such enthusiasm from the word go, and everyone at St. Martin's Press who supported this project throughout. It really makes a difference knowing you have a whole publishing house cheering you on!

This couldn't have happened without the support and understanding of our family and friends who helped us make it through all the blood (ahem), sweat, and tears.

Last, our tremendous thanks to the many women who thoughtfully answered our questions about their embarrassing, hilarious, scary, curious, confusing, frustrating, and gleeful experiences with menstruation and menopause.

About the Authors

ELISSA STEIN is a published author whose work includes visual histories of iconic pop culture, New York City adventures with kids, and interactive thank-you notes. In addition to writing, she runs her own graphic design business. To balance the above, she practices yoga, knits with enthusiasm, and collects vintage coats. She lives in New York City with her husband, Jon, and their children, Izzy and Jack.

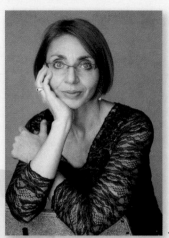

Frank Veronsky

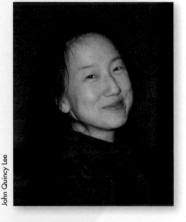

John Quincy Lee

As a playwright, **SUSAN KIM** wrote the stage adaptation of *The Joy Luck Club* (Dramatists Play Service) and numerous one-acts, which have been produced widely. She is a Writers Guild award-winning TV writer in documentary and children's programming, and has been nominated five times for the Emmy. With her boyfriend, novelist and playwright Laurence Klavan, she wrote two graphic novels, *Circle of Spies* and *The Fielding Course* (First Second Books). She teaches dramatic writing in the MFA program of Goddard College and lives in New York City with Klavan.